Heal Your Love-Hate Relationship with Food

AN INTUITIVE EATING & INTERNAL FAMILY SYSTEMS WORKBOOK

KIMBERLY M. DANIELS, PsyD

New Harbinger Publications, Inc.

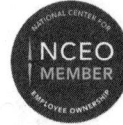

Cover design by Amy Shoup

Acquired by Jed Bickman

Edited by Karen Schader

Library of Congress Cataloging-in-Publication Data on file

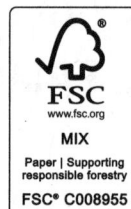

Printed in the United States of America

28   27   26

10 9 8 7 6 5 4 3 2 1   First Printing

"As I read Kim Daniels's book, I imagined my inner eating system sitting under a beautiful tree, with my Self present, listening, as each part reflected on how it was impacted by one of the principles of Intuitive Eating: unconditional permission to eat. Daniels's integration of Internal Family Systems (IFS) and Intuitive Eating is gentle, as she takes the reader's hand and guides them through this healing work."

—**Tammy Sollenberger, LCMHC**, author of *The One Inside*

"Kim Daniels does a beautiful job explaining the IFS model and how it can be helpful in developing a more compassionate relationship with food. In her easy-to-read writing style and her reflective writing exercises, Kim helps the reader gain insight, understanding, and self-compassion."

—**Sue Richmond, LCSW**, IFS Lead Trainer

"Who doesn't need help finding peace with food? Using a dynamite combination of IFS and Intuitive Eating principles, Kim Daniels has written a smart, user-friendly guide to help us get to know and find peace with the conflicting inner voices we carry when it comes to food, chronic dieting, and body image. I know that's a mouthful—just get the book! Your parts will thank you."

—**Colleen West, LMFT**, author of *We All Have Parts* and *The Internal Family Systems (IFS) Flip Chart*

"Kim Daniels is a compassionate and no-nonsense guide to getting to know and healing your eating parts using IFS. Daniels offers clear direction for relearning eating skills, using the principles of Intuitive Eating integrated into parts work. This book is a road map for anyone who wants to calm the chaos around food in their minds and bodies, and eat in a self-led way."

—**Cinnamon Holsclaw, LCSW**, Certified IFS Therapist

"This is a comprehensive workbook that incorporates the most salient principles of IFS and Intuitive Eating into one valuable toolkit. This is a great resource for anyone who has been suffering from diet culture, disordered eating, and body-image issues. As a therapist who works in this specialty area, I see this workbook being very helpful to many individuals who struggle with these issues. I highly recommend it!"

—**Elizabeth I. Rathbun, PsyD, CEDS**, Certified Intuitive Eating Counselor and clinical psychologist in private practice

For my daughter, Jillian—you're my favorite and my best.

Contents

Introduction

"I have a love-hate relationship with food." I can't tell you how many times I've heard these words from clients. This short, simple sentence summarizes how many view food, but it cannot remotely convey the complexity of their relationship with it.

Most of us have a complicated relationship with food. When you think about it, this relationship began the day you were born. (Actually, probably even before. What your biological mother ate and how responsive she was to her hunger during pregnancy likely impacted your connection to food.) Indeed, your relationship with food is one of the few relationships you've had throughout your entire life. And it's gone through many iterations, I'm sure. You may have been a toddler who ate only chicken nuggets, and progressed to a little kid who ate only grilled cheese, and then moved on to become an adult who eats anything on their plate. You may have gone through a vegetarian phase, a vegan phase, a carnivore phase. Maybe those phases turned into a sustained eating pattern, or maybe they fell by the wayside.

Your relationship with food could very well have included dieting, as an estimated 45 million Americans go on a diet each year. You may be someone who has tried one diet or what feels like a million different diets (or the same one eighteen times). And how you relate to food probably changed with each one you tried. Likely, you counted something (calories, points, carbohydrates); weighed and measured your food; or cut out certain foods or food groups. Different foods were probably considered "good" or "bad," given whatever plan you were on, and some foods may have been completely demonized.

Food is a huge part of our lives. It's something that we see, touch, smell, taste, and consume daily (hopefully), most likely multiple times per day. Hours are spent shopping for, preparing, cooking, and consuming food each week. We socialize with food, talk about our day over food, and nurture others with food. And sometimes we comfort ourselves with it.

In addition to your relationship with food being lifelong, it's been shaped by multiple factors, the most prominent being your family. How we view food is heavily influenced by how our caregivers viewed food. They're the ones who chose the foods we tended to eat—at least until we were old enough to choose our own—portioned out our food, taught us to cook, and possibly even introduced us to dieting.

(*Note:* Parents are the primary caregivers for many of us, so going forward, I'll use the word "parent." Please mentally substitute "caregiver" if that fits your family.)

How you view food has also been influenced by your friends, peers, and significant others. It's been further shaped by the many cultural circles you've lived in: your ethnic culture, your religious culture, and perhaps even your work culture.

Your relationship with food has also been heavily influenced by one of the biggest cultures in the United States (and other countries): diet culture. None of us has escaped diet culture. It's impossible. Diet culture is everywhere. Hardly anyone can go one day without seeing ads for diet programs, weight-loss medication, or diet pills. You cannot browse your local bookstore without seeing diet cookbooks. And you probably cannot even have a night out with your family and friends without someone mentioning their latest weight-loss attempt or making negative comments about their own body.

All of us have had a long relationship with food. And for many of us, that relationship is difficult. My guess is that since you've picked up this book, you're struggling with yours. And if that's the case, I'm so glad you're here.

I'd also wager that this isn't the first book about eating that you've read or started to read. And since you've picked up yet another book, you probably didn't find the answers you were looking for in the others. I can only imagine your frustration.

You might be really skeptical about this book too. Will this one be helpful? Does this author know what she's talking about? Does she know my experience? Will I find myself in these pages? Will I finish this book and think, *I finally figured it out?*

I feel pretty strongly that the answer to those questions will be yes.

Who This Book Is For

This workbook is for anyone who struggles with food. It's for those who say they have a love-hate relationship with food and for anyone who describes food as their best friend and their worst enemy. It's for those who say, "I'm an emotional eater," "a comfort eater," "a binge eater," or "a stress eater."

This book is for those who say, "I eat for all the wrong reasons. And I have no idea why." And for those who say, "I *know* why I eat. I just can't stop." It's for you if you've ever denied yourself your favorite food because you "shouldn't" have it, eaten in the dark for fear of being seen, numbed your feelings with a bag of chips, or stopped at a drive-through on your way home from a stressful workday only to later eat a full meal with your family so no one notices.

This workbook is also for you if you've been on one diet or twenty-seven. Or if you've jumped from plan to plan, desperate to find the one that works. It's for anyone who's ever thought, *I failed again*. (No, you didn't. But we'll get to that later.) And if you've ever felt the shame of regaining your lost weight (and possibly additional weight), this book is for you too.

This workbook is also for those who have ever felt not good enough because of their body. Those who have been told their body is unhealthy, unworthy, wrong. It's for anyone who went to their physician for a sinus infection and was given a pamphlet on semaglutide drugs for weight loss or bariatric surgery. And it's even for you if you've taken medication or had bariatric surgery and didn't find the answer you were promised and were desperately hoping for.

If any of this resonates with you, you're not alone. But you may be wondering how in the world one workbook could be that helpful to such a large audience.

As a psychologist who specializes in food and body concerns, I've helped countless clients with the skills included in this book, and I've seen these skills work wonders. From those with diagnosable eating disorders to those who are just frustrated that they can't get a handle on their relationship with food, I've seen people make huge shifts in their eating patterns and in how they feel about their body by using the skills I'm going to teach you.

I truly believe that these approaches will work for you too. That's why I wrote this book.

The approaches to healing your relationship with food and your body that you'll find in this book are powerful, but not instant. The skills and concepts aren't magical, and they aren't even all that complicated. But they take commitment, thought, and the willingness to truly get to know yourself. It starts and ends with being able to connect with and sit with yourself.

That's not always easy. But I believe you can do it.

I also know that what you've been doing isn't easy either: jumping from diet to diet; feeling out of control with food; telling yourself *Tomorrow I'll start over*; hating your body. None of that is easy. In fact, I think it's far more difficult than what you'll find in the pages of this book.

My guess is that by this point, you might be feeling a mix of emotions. Maybe anxiety that you're about to look at food in a different way, skepticism that this book will actually help you, and even excitement that perhaps it will. All of these feelings are normal. Digging into your relationship with food and your body always brings up a number of feelings. And they're all valid, so remember to notice them.

Let's Talk About Weight Loss

You might also be wondering if this book will help you lose weight. This question is in the background of almost every conversation about emotional eating, overeating, binge eating, and obviously, dieting. Because at the heart of wanting to change your eating patterns is almost always a desire to change your body. Very often, it's *all* about wanting to change your body. So let's talk about that.

First and foremost, this is not a weight-loss book. And the more you read, the more you'll understand why focusing on weight loss isn't helpful and, in fact, often leads to weight *gain*. It also tends to lead to the eating behaviors you're trying to stop, such as binge eating, overeating, and emotional eating. Focusing on weight loss also supports the notion given to us by diet culture—that our weight defines us. That if we're thin, we're acceptable, but if we're large, we're not. I don't believe that and have no desire to support that, and I don't want you to either. And finally, focusing on weight loss takes the emphasis off the things about you that are so much more important than your size, like your interests, your personality, and the qualities that make you *you*. Those have *nothing* to do with your weight.

Having said all of that, though, I completely understand if you're someone who wants to lose weight. It's not easy, or always safe, to be in a large body in the US and many other countries. Many aspects of our society are not designed for large bodies. Airline seats. Restaurant booths. Waiting room chairs. Roller coasters. Our medical community has taken on the message of diet culture and is emphatic that large bodies are never healthy—and that is *not* true. And let's not forget that people in large bodies are consistently stigmatized, marginalized, and oppressed.

If you're hoping that this book will help you lose weight, I completely understand that hope. Will it? I have no idea. I would never promise you that your body will change because I cannot know that. No one can.

But I can tell you that weight loss is not achievable with what you're doing now. As you'll read in chapter 7, dieting fails almost 100 percent of the time. Whatever you're doing now is not going to lead to sustained weight loss. Working on your relationship with food and your body is your best chance. Regardless of what we are consistently told by diet culture and our medical community, not all bodies are meant to be small. And only about 20–30 percent of our weight is determined by what we eat and how we move. The rest is a mix of genetics and social factors, such as income level, access to health care, and even your zip code.

No, I will not guarantee you or anyone else weight loss. But one of my hopes for you is that by the end of this workbook, you won't care so much about your weight anyway. At the very least, I hope you'll come to respect your body and treat it with kindness, no matter its size.

At this point, I encourage you to reflect on what you've read thus far. What thoughts are you having? What feelings? What are you noticing in your body?

_____

_____

_____

_____

_____

_____

_____

Who Am I to Help You?

I believe it's extremely important that you know who I am and why I chose to write this book. I'm a clinical psychologist who has been working with people who struggle with food and body concerns for over twenty years. And I spent about fifteen years of that time doing it all wrong.

For years, while working in a bariatric surgery program, I helped my clients focus on weight loss. And sure, sometimes clients lost weight, improved their health, and lived out happy, fulfilled lives. But other times, clients regained their lost weight, redeveloped the health issues they thought had been resolved with weight loss, and experienced depression and feelings of hopelessness because life wasn't what they thought it would be like following their surgery.

Even those who maintained their weight loss struggled. Many experienced extremely negative body images and felt worse about their bodies than they had previously. Many who lost weight and maintained their loss also dealt with extreme anxiety about potential weight regain and were never quite able to enjoy life because of this.

As I noticed these issues with so many postoperative patients, I started changing how I worked with them. I moved away from the focus on weight loss and toward a Health at Every Size (HAES) framework. It was through researching HAES that I found Intuitive Eating (IE) (Tribole and Resch 2020), one of the approaches I'll be discussing later in the book. I then began incorporating Internal

Family Systems (IFS), another model I'll be sharing with you in this book. This game-changing combination of IFS and IE has been highly effective in helping my clients truly heal their relationships with food and their bodies, and I'm so excited to introduce it to you.

One last thing that I think is very important for you to know: I do not live in a large body, and I never have. If you're someone in a large body who is now doubting my ability to help you, I understand that. I leave it up to you to make the choice of whether to continue reading. I've worked with numerous clients over the years who live in large bodies, and I have tremendous compassion for those people who are marginalized for any reason. Despite that, I'm well aware that merely working with these clients isn't the same as having a lived experience. Regardless, I still believe that the approaches we discuss in this book can be invaluable to you. I hope you give them a chance.

How to Use This Book

The skills in this book are meant to build upon each other, so I strongly suggest starting at chapter 1 and working through the chapters in sequence. At http://www.newharbinger.com, you'll also find free tools that you can download.

Please be patient with yourself. Some of the concepts presented will likely resonate with you immediately, while others may not. Similarly, some of the exercises you'll be doing will take more time, thought, and effort than others. That's okay. Have no expectation for yourself in terms of how soon you'll complete the book. The adage I'd like you to remember is: "It takes as long as it takes."

If you're working with a therapist, coach, or other helping professional, consider taking the book into that work. Having the support of another helper would most likely provide additional insight. Sharing the book and the work you're doing with a safe person who can support you may also be helpful.

If you aren't currently seeing a helping professional and you find that the book is bringing up distressing thoughts, beliefs, and emotions, put it down, and consider seeking help. Although some of this work may be uncomfortable, it should in no way be incapacitating. Similarly, if you're struggling with a diagnosed eating disorder, have a history of untreated trauma, or have been diagnosed with a dissociative disorder, *please do not use this book without the help of a trained therapist*. And finally, please know that this book is not a substitute for therapy. If you're in need of a trained professional, look at the list of resources at the end of the book.

Checking In

These questions are designed to guide you toward a deeper understanding of yourself and where you are currently. You'll find many of these types of questions throughout the book. Please take your time to reflect on and respond to them, and refer back to them from time to time to add any new thoughts and insights that come up.

How would you describe your current relationship with food?

_____

_____

_____

_____

How would you like that to change?

_____

_____

_____

How would you describe your current relationship with your body?

_____

_____

_____

_____

How would you like that to change?

_____

_____

_____

What are you hoping to learn or accomplish with the help of this book?

_____

_____

_____

_____

_____

_____

CHAPTER 1

A New Approach

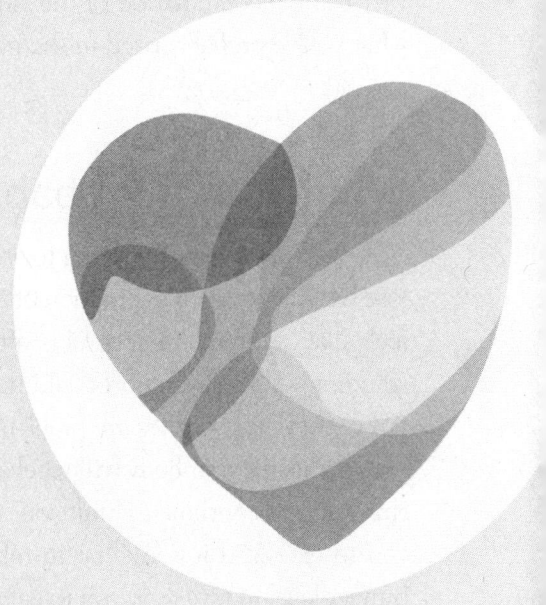

As you read in the introduction, this workbook will teach you how to use IFS and IE to heal your relationships with food and your body. This is the game-changing combination that I've seen work countless times with clients. In this chapter, I'm going to tell you a little more about IFS and IE and why using a combination of the two is so incredibly helpful. But before that, let's quickly talk about what you've probably tried in the past and why it didn't work.

What You've Probably Tried and Why It Didn't Work

Whether you were attempting to end your emotional eating, stop bingeing, gain control over food, or lose weight (or any combination of these), you likely used restriction to achieve your goals. Restriction feels like control, and control is often the goal (although it really shouldn't be—control isn't understanding). This restriction could have come in the form of dieting, medication, or bariatric surgery. All of those approaches are problematic for both physical and emotional reasons.

Physically, your body will rebel against restriction because it doesn't want to die. And that's a good thing! If you continue to limit your food intake, your body will kick in and do whatever it can to force you to eat. And it does that in really cool ways, like turning on the hormones that ramp up your hunger level to try to get you to eat; lowering the hormones that tell your body you're full so you'll eat more; expanding what your taste buds enjoy in order to get you to eat anything at all. Yes, restriction often *leads* to eating.

Emotionally, restriction is problematic because *food is comforting and enjoyable.* We can pass by our favorite foods for only so long before we say, "Enough! I don't care anymore. I want the damn cookies!" That's *normal.* That's not a lack of willpower or a lack of control. It's *normal* to enjoy food and to want to eat foods we like. We cannot sustain depriving ourselves of these foods long-term.

In addition to our enjoying food, it is a huge comfort to many of us. My guess is, if I asked you to make a list of your comfort foods, you would immediately start naming items like chocolate chip cookies. Ice cream. A warm mug of hot cocoa. Anything with cheese. *Food is comforting*, and we *all* need comfort.

Food is also an amazing distraction. It's been my experience that one of the main reasons people turn to food is to distract themselves from difficult emotions. And food is *really* good for that. It's delicious, enjoyable, and hopefully readily available. And if you're using food that way, restricting it can become nearly impossible because you suddenly don't have a distraction. Now that the food is gone, those feelings it was helping you avoid are front and center.

And finally, one of the biggest reasons that dieting, surgery, and medication don't help your emotional eating is because none of them in any way, shape, or form help you understand *why* you're using food the way you are. These methods are all about changing and controlling behavior. They aren't about understanding it. And behavior change without understanding doesn't work.

IFS and IE: A Game-Changing Combination

I'm going to repeat that point: behavior change by itself, without understanding, doesn't work. I cannot say this enough. In order to make a change in your eating patterns, you *must* understand why you use or restrict food. And there's no better way to help you understand this than IFS.

Next, we're going to talk about what IFS and IE are and how the combination of these approaches is different than anything you've tried in the past.

What Is IFS?

Quick question: have you ever seen the movie *Inside Out*? It's a fantastic Pixar movie where we see five parts who make up the mind of the main character, Riley. This movie is a great example of the core tenet of IFS: our minds are made up of subpersonalities, or parts. Each part has a certain role to play in what we call our internal system, and all of our parts are trying to be helpful to us. Sometimes our parts use or restrict food in order to be helpful. For example, if you are someone who tends to eat in order to zone out when you're stressed, that means a *part* of you uses food to help distract you. Or, if you tend to feel the need to fit in well with others, you may have a *part* who uses dieting to do that.

In addition to parts, IFS holds that we also have a core Self, which is considered to be our authentic self, or our true essence. Our Self is a wonderful resource for our parts and embodies such qualities as compassion, curiosity, calmness, and confidence.

In this book, you'll be getting to know the parts of you who relate to food in various ways, and you'll learn how to access your true Self. This understanding will allow you to approach your parts, your body, and food in a much more calm, curious way, which will lead to healing your relationships with food and your body. All of this paves the way to using the skills of IE.

What Is IE?

Intuitive Eating (IE) is a model created by Evelyn Tribole and Elyse Resch (2020), dietitians who both recognized that the typical way of approaching food and nutrition (that is, counting calories, weighing and measuring food, focusing on weight loss) wasn't working for their clients. At least not in the long run. So they dove into the research and developed their own model that aims to help you stop dieting, eat foods that you enjoy, no longer fear food, and respect your body.

IE includes ten principles that help you achieve these goals:

1.   Reject diet culture

2.   Honor your hunger

3.   Make peace with food

4.   Discover the satisfaction factor

5.   Feel your fullness

6.   Challenge the food police

7.   Cope with your emotions with kindness

8.   Respect your body

9.   Movement—feel the difference

10.   Honor your health—gentle nutrition

The main goal of IE is *attunement*: the ability to tune into your body and recognize what it needs. When you're able to do that, you can eat in ways that are satisfying. You will no longer eat to the point of discomfort (at least not regularly), and you'll eat foods that feel good to your body. You'll be able to eat your "fear foods" when you like *and* without having to work them into a calorie count.

How This Approach Is Different

As you read earlier, IFS is the best way I've ever found to truly understand why you relate to food the way you do. With IFS, you'll get to know the specific parts of you who eat for various reasons and those who restrict food. You'll literally ask the parts themselves why they do what they do. And guess what—they'll tell you! You don't have to surmise or guess why they're doing what they're doing—you'll just ask them. And you'll develop a relationship with those parts that will eventually allow them to shift what they're doing.

With the help of IFS, you'll also come to understand that the parts of you who eat when you're upset, who binge eat, who can't seem to stop dieting *are all trying to be helpful to you*. For most people, this is a very different way of looking at their eating patterns. Most of us are extremely hard on ourselves, especially when it comes to our bodies and our eating habits. We tend to be critical and even angry at ourselves. That isn't at all helpful. You can't hate yourself into changing.

Instead, with the help of IFS, you'll be approaching your parts—and your body—with compassion, curiosity, and calmness. Take a moment to imagine how that might feel, and jot some notes here:

_____

_____

_____

_____

_____

_____

With the understanding and self-compassion that IFS provides as your base, you'll then be able to use the principles of IE to help you stop restricting food and eat the food you enjoy. You'll be capable of tuning into your body, noticing your hunger and fullness cues, and nourishing it in the ways it wants and needs. Finally, you'll develop trust in the wisdom of your Self and your body, leading you to approach food with calm awareness and intention.

That may sound like a lot of concepts and lofty ideas, so let's talk about what will actually change for you. With the help of IFS and IE, you will:

develop a deep understanding of why you use food the way you do;

no longer diet or restrict your food intake;

be able to keep your "fear foods" at home without bingeing on them;

feel at ease with food and no longer need to control it;

treat your body with kindness and respect;

eat in a way that serves your body well;

respond to your body's hunger and fullness cues; and

regularly enjoy the food you love without feeling guilt or shame.

And you'll know within your bones that your body is your home, and it's good enough just the way it is.

Why This Approach Can Be Scary

Right now, you may have a lot of different feelings. There may be parts of you who are thrilled at the thought of never dieting again, or of eating the foods you love and have been avoiding, and who are ready to jump into the car right now to go buy M&Ms. You may have parts who can't wait to understand why you use food the way you do, to stop binge eating, or to stop leaning on food for emotional reasons.

But I'm guessing you also have parts who are feeling terrified. Terrified of giving up your latest or favorite diet. Or your favorite food. Scared of potentially gaining weight. Fearful of failing at this new approach. And fearful of succeeding at it too.

These fears are completely understandable, especially if you're someone who's been dieting or eating in response to your emotions for most of your life. The thought of trying something new—and possibly something you've never even heard of before—is daunting. And again, that's completely understandable.

So let's talk about it, starting with the fear of no longer dieting. This can be scary for a number of reasons. Not dieting means listening to yourself in terms of food. It means checking in with your body and understanding what it needs. That's *very* scary for my clients. They typically say, "But I won't know what to eat!" Which makes sense, given that they've always just eaten what someone else has told them to eat. It's very scary to think about basing your food decisions on what your body is telling you to eat.

What we're talking about here is trust. Diet culture has consistently told all of us that we can't trust ourselves around food. That if left to our own devices, we'll all be bingeing in front of the fridge on a daily basis. The culture has created this fear. And this fear is completely unfounded.

From birth, all of us have the ability to tune into our bodies and know how and what to eat. Think about infants and toddlers. They eat when they're hungry, they stop when they're full (sometimes quite dramatically by throwing their food on the floor), and they know what they want to eat. You were born with that ability, and you can return to it.

If you're afraid of gaining weight as a result of this new approach, that's understandable as well. Again, large bodies are treated very differently than small bodies. It makes sense that some parts worry about gaining weight and how that might impact your life, your relationships, and your view of yourself.

The fear of potentially losing food as your emotional coping skill is scary as well. Very often, my clients say something like, "Food is the only thing I have." Giving it up is terrifying. But I want to reassure you that the goal here is *not* giving up food as a comfort. That's not realistic, and it's not necessary. You can still turn to food when you need to. You'll just be able to do it in a much calmer, more aware manner.

I get that all of this is scary. And before moving on, you'll be noticing and reflecting on the fears you have about moving forward with this book. I encourage you to take all of this at your own pace. There is no need to rush. These concepts take time to really sink in and digest (pardon the pun). Slow and steady wins the race here.

And I encourage you to keep moving forward with this work. You deserve peace, ease, and freedom with food and your body. You can have all of that if you keep going.

Checking In

Take some time to reflect on the following questions. Notice any thoughts, feelings, or bodily sensations that arise when you consider these questions, and write about them in the space provided.

What are the fears you have about learning a new approach to food? To your body?

_____

_____

_____

_____

_____

_____

What concerns do you have about diving deeper into your relationship with food and your body?

_____

_____

_____

_____

_____

What have you done in the past to try to address your eating patterns?

_____

_____

_____

_____

What were those attempts like for you? What did you like about what you were trying? What didn't you like?

_____

_____

_____

_____

What were your typical results?

_____

_____

_____

If these attempts weren't successful, how did you feel when they didn't work?

_____

_____

_____

Looking back at it, did you blame yourself when they didn't work? If so, what's your reaction to my saying "It *wasn't* your fault"?

_____

_____

_____

_____

CHAPTER 2

IFS and Your Eating Parts

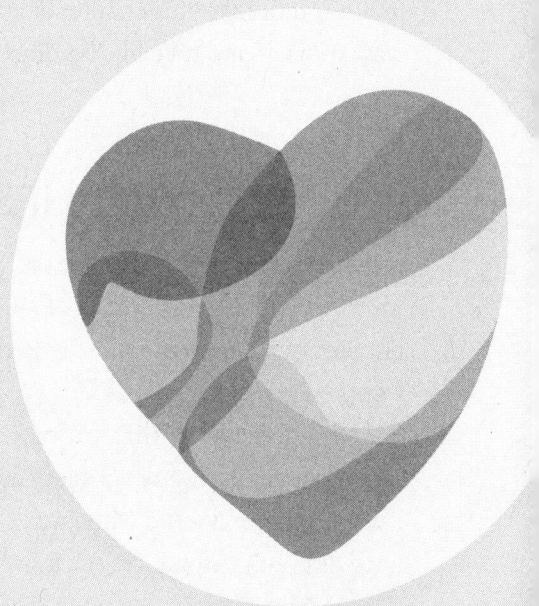

In chapter 1, I gave you a brief intro to IFS and how it can be helpful. In this chapter, we're going to go into the details of the model as well as looking at common parts many people have regarding food. There will be ample opportunities for you to notice your own parts and reflect on what you read. I invite you to take this chapter at your own pace—it may be a lot to take in at first glance! Be patient with yourself and take all the time you need.

A Deep Dive Into IFS

Have you ever heard yourself say, "Part of me wants that, but part of me doesn't"? Or "Part of me wants that cupcake, but part of me thinks it's bad for me." Or "Part of me wants to take that new job, but part of me is terrified!" Or "Part of me says I should go out and be social, but part of me really just wants to stay home."

My guess is now that you're thinking about it, you're realizing you've done this before. Probably numerous times. I've never met anyone who hasn't. We all talk in the language of parts without even thinking about it. And when we do that, we're supporting the fundamental tenet of IFS: that we don't have just one personality, one mind. We're all multiple, meaning we have many different subpersonalities, or "parts."

I know that may seem a little out there (or maybe it doesn't; some people resonate with this idea instantly), but it makes so much sense when you think about it. The idea of multiplicity explains why we have so many different thoughts and feelings about the same person, situation, event, and so on: we literally have different parts of us who carry these varying thoughts and feelings.

Just a little background on how IFS was created before we get into the details. The model was founded by Dr. Richard Schwartz over thirty years ago. While working with clients diagnosed with bulimia, Dr. Schwartz began noticing his clients talking about parts (Schwartz 1995). They would say things like: "A part of me wants to stop bingeing, but another part of me doesn't." He became very curious about this and realized that he himself had parts. He eventually combined his knowledge of family systems theory with this idea of parts and created a model that views individuals as having their own internal family system (hence the name).

Let's flesh this idea out a bit with a brief exercise. I invite you to think of an important person in your life. Someone you truly love and care about. Take a moment to think about this person, and then write down all the different feelings you have toward them. Here's an example:

Person: *My daughter*

Feelings: *Love, respect, compassion, pride, awe, overwhelmed, worry for her present and future, more love, frustration*

Now you try it:

Person: _____

Feelings: _____

_____

_____

_____

Do you see how you don't have just one feeling toward that person? You have many different feelings. And those feelings are likely different parts, each carrying their own feeling. Looking at my example, of course I love my daughter more than anyone. But I have parts who are overwhelmed by having been a single parent for so long. I also have parts who are anxious about the world she's living in. When she goes off to college, I will no doubt have parts who are immensely excited for her, as well as parts who miss her terribly. And I'll have parts who are *so glad* to have the house to myself! These are all different parts with different feelings toward and about her. My guess is that your list is similar, with your feelings ranging from one end of the spectrum to the other.

Let's look at another example: how you feel toward food. We've been talking about how complicated our relationship with food is, and part of that complexity is a result of having multiple parts with many different feelings about and experiences with food.

Take a moment to write down all the different feelings you have toward food:

_____

_____

_____

_____

_____

Most likely, your feelings ran from love to hate and made various stops in between. This is because you have numerous parts who have different ideas about, reactions to, and uses for food. We'll be exploring all those parts in this book.

What Are Parts?

Parts, again, are little subpersonalities within our personality. They each have a different role in our system, with parts taking over or "driving the bus" at different times, depending on what's going on. When a part is running the show, we say that we are blended with that part. That means that the part has essentially taken control of the wheel, and our thoughts, feelings, and behaviors are coming from that part.

We're almost always blended with our parts throughout the day, and this is completely normal. We have parts who do our jobs well, parent our kids, know their way around town, and engage in fun activities. You likely have dozens of parts who are keeping your life running, and you don't necessarily need to do anything about them. The ones we'll be concentrating on in this book are the ones who are highly focused on food, on what you eat or don't eat, who restrict food, and who are focused on your body's appearance and possibly wanting to change it. We'll especially focus on the parts who impulsively and strongly take over your eating process. We call that being "hijacked" by a part. You may resonate with that word, as sometimes you may feel that you aren't even present when you're eating. It's like someone else took over and ate half the pantry in your absence. These very strong parts become so quickly and easily blended with us that they control our every move. We don't even have the space from them to think about what we're doing. My guess is that happens to you with food sometimes (or a lot of the time). We'll be talking about how to approach these parts later in the book.

Everyone experiences their parts differently. Some people can see their parts, some can't. Some peoples' parts are visible but are not necessarily in human form. They're animals, shapes, or other objects. Others don't see their parts, but they hear them, or just have a felt-sense of them. There's no right or wrong way to experience your parts. For me, all my parts (those I've met so far) look like separate people. Some of them look like me at various ages, and many of them look very different from me. Some identify as male, some as female, some as neither.

Our parts fall into one of two categories: exiles or protectors. Let's take a closer look at these different roles.

Exiles

Exiles are the parts of us who carry extreme beliefs and emotions (in IFS, we call these "burdens") that have resulted from trauma and other difficult life experiences. They tend to be young parts who are truly hurting and are stuck in the past where the damage was done. Our systems tend to exile these parts (or push them underground) because we cannot function well when they take over, as they tend to flood us with emotions.

There are a few common themes in the burdens exiles carry. Many carry feelings or beliefs of unworthiness, low self-worth, inadequacy, and shame. You may also have parts who carry significant sadness, loneliness, and fear. The emotions and beliefs your exiles carry depend upon your life experiences, and none of us have exactly the same parts.

All of us have exiles. You may be noticing some of yours making themselves known right now. I'd like for those parts to know that they aren't alone, and that there is hope for feeling better.

I invite you to list any exiles you're noticing now:

_____

_____

_____

Protectors

Because we're largely ineffective, if not incapacitated, when our exiles take over and flood our system, we have protector parts who jump in to either make them feel better or to exile them even more (that is, to push them underground in order to quiet them or protect them from getting hurt again). There are two types of protector parts: managers and firefighters.

Managers are proactive, organized, and on top of things. They're the parts of us who are responsible and get things done. Managers also try to control other people and events, and even other parts. They protect against anything that leads to vulnerability, pain, or instability. In relation to food and your body, manager parts are, for example, those who

prep meals;

stick to exactly what's on your grocery list;

count calories;

weigh and measure food; and

weigh yourself regularly.

Firefighters, on the other hand, are reactive, impulsive, and extreme. They're literally there to put out the flames of intense feeling. They swoop in to numb or soothe whatever discomfort your parts are experiencing. Firefighters act automatically to repress whatever it is that your exiles are feeling. They tend to engage in extreme behaviors, like substance abuse, self-injury, and binge eating. If you've ever binged, you may recall feeling as if you were in a trance or a food coma. This is exactly what your binge eating part wants: for you to feel nothing.

Firefighters also jump in in reaction to food restriction. They're tired of being restricted by others around you (for example, a partner who doesn't allow you to eat sugar), your own managers who are trying to protect you with restriction, and diet culture at large. In response to that, they lead you to binge or eat compulsively.

Examples of firefighters are parts who

binge;

use food to soothe or distract you;

steer you into a fast-food restaurant without thinking;

engage in purging behaviors, like vomiting or excessive exercise;

desperately start yet another diet; or

start a weight-loss medication or schedule a bariatric surgery consultation without giving them much consideration.

The protective parts in our system are always trying to do just that: protect us. They're here to help us. They have all taken on certain jobs based on their experiences, and they continue to do these jobs in the same way until they feel safe or comfortable enough to do them differently or not at all. Our parts don't jump from job to job. The parts of you who lead you to food don't suddenly become the parts who organize your kitchen cabinets. They will remain the parts leading you to food until you help them either let go of their jobs or change them.

By this point, you may be thinking, *These parts are trying to help? Are you kidding me? I hate what they're doing!* I completely understand that. These are often the parts the field of psychiatry labels as symptoms or disorders that we must treat and fix. These are the parts our society deems wrong that we want to just get rid of.

Emotional eating is a great example of this. Every client I've ever seen who describes themselves as an emotional eater has come to me wanting to stop this behavior. Using food for comfort, stress relief, as a reward, and so on has been vilified in our society (and to some degree by the field of psychiatry). We're supposed to end this practice, but the parts of us who are using food for these reasons *truly* believe that they're helping us. They absolutely believe that food is the thing that will fix whatever is happening in that moment.

Knowing the difference between managers and firefighters isn't always necessary, and sometimes it's not that easy to distinguish between the two. Sometimes I can't even tell if my clients' parts are managers or firefighters. It's really just important to know that we have protective parts. Having said that, I'll offer this little explanation that I learned from one of my trainers. Let's say you're going to a social event and you're someone who tends to get a little anxious at these types of outings. Your manager parts may lead you to have a glass of wine prior to the event in order to calm your nerves. But let's say you get to the party and your anxious parts really take over. Your firefighters may lead you to have a bottle of wine at the event in order to numb your nerves. Managers are proactive and anticipate difficulties; firefighters are reactive and extreme.

One last thing about firefighters. If your firefighters are leading you to engage in daily episodes of binge eating, purging behaviors, or severe restriction, please seek help from an eating disorder therapist as soon as possible. These behaviors are beyond the scope of this book and need to be addressed with an experienced professional.

Characteristics of Parts

Here are a few more things to know about parts before we move along:

Parts are often stuck in time. When difficult or traumatic events occur, our parts often remain stuck in that time period. It's like they picked up their burdens and weren't able to leave. This concept actually helps explain a few things, the first being why we don't always feel like the grown-ups we are. Have you ever felt like you are much younger than you are? Like when you're with your family? This is because your child or teenage parts, who are stuck in the past, are running the show at these times.

The idea that our parts are stuck in time also explains why they can become retraumatized so easily. Our parts can truly believe they're back in the situation that created the burden. They have no idea that those days are long gone, and they're constantly reliving the trauma. You may have noticed that you sometimes respond to current events with more emotion than seems warranted. This is because it's not the current experience that's triggering your parts. It's something from the past that was traumatic to a younger part of you who had few skills or resources to manage it.

Let's look at an example. If you experienced the trauma of bullying as a child, it's extremely likely that you still have at least one young part (who's the same age as when the bullying happened) who has no idea that that experience has long since passed. This part still expects to be traumatized, even though you're no longer a child facing a bully. The part believes that danger is still present. This may explain why you might be really nervous in social situations or you may not like large groups. That poor little part is terrified that you're going to be bullied again.

Parts don't know how old we are. Many of our parts have no idea of our current age and no concept that there's a grown-up around (your Self) who can take care of them. Because of this, we have parts trying to do jobs that they're much too young to do. I've found that many people with food and body concerns have young parts who needed to be overly responsible during their childhood, and they've carried this responsibility into adulthood. These parts still believe that there's no adult present who can be helpful to them, when in fact there is—your Self. Therefore, one of the things we do regularly in IFS is let our parts know our current age and our current life circumstances. We call this updating.

Many parts don't know other parts. Our parts don't all know each other, even if they're all in the same system. Some of them have met before; others have had the experience of being completely alone their entire lives.

Before we continue, take a moment to notice how your parts are responding to this information.

What is your reaction to the idea that you're a system made up of parts?

_____

_____

_____

_____

When you think about yourself in terms of parts, what thoughts, feelings, and bodily sensations do you notice?

_____

_____

_____

_____

What is it like for you to consider that your relationship with food is adaptive (that is, the parts who lead you to eat or to restrict are actually trying to help)?

_____

_____

_____

_____

What Is the Self?

In addition to parts, we all have a Self, which is our core essence (some people call it their higher self, higher power, authentic me, or soul). This was another of Dr. Schwartz's insights. As he became more and more curious about his clients' parts, he often heard them say something like, "That doesn't feel like a part. That feels like me." He began referring to this as the Self (Schwartz 1995). It's who we truly are.

Dr. Schwartz began noticing that each person's Self had similar qualities. And conveniently, they all started with the letter C. We refer to these as the 8 C's:

- Compassion

- Curiosity

- Calmness

- Confidence

- Clarity

- Connectedness

- Creativity

- Courage

In IFS, we talk about being "in Self," having "Self-energy," or being "Self-led," meaning that we're connected to and embodying at least one of the 8 C's. We don't need to embody all eight in order to be in Self—that would be really difficult! But even connecting to just one of those qualities brings Self-energy to our parts and to those around us.

At this point, you may be wondering if you have a Self. And the answer is a resounding yes! But again, our Self tends to be blended with parts much of the time. Regardless, like the sun, your Self is always there, even when you can't see it. Building trust between your Self and your parts is a big part of the process in IFS, and we'll be starting that process in the next chapter.

Before continuing, take a moment to respond to the prompts on the following page.

What is your reaction to the idea that you have a Self, an inner resource who's always there for your parts?

_____

_____

_____

_____

Which of the 8 C's do you feel you access most easily?

_____

_____

_____

Think of times when you are in Self. What does that feel like for you? (If you're having a difficult time with this, that's okay. We'll be practicing this in the next chapter.)

_____

_____

_____

_____

Your Eating System

Within our internal family system of parts, we have what I call an eating system. This is a subsystem of all the parts who have anything to do with food and your body. It includes, but is not limited to, parts who love food, who use food for comfort, who restrict food, and who have feelings about your body. These parts either relate to each other in different ways, or don't relate to each other at all.

Some of our parts work together and have the same goals. You may have parts who work together to start you on the next diet, keep you going on the one you started months ago, or keep you focused on weight loss in other ways. Similarly, you may have parts who work together to make sure you always have your favorite snacks in the house. Or who support other parts in eating whatever they want.

Some of our parts, however, really don't like each other. If you have a binge eating part, you probably have parts who don't like it. They don't like how you feel physically after bingeing, they feel shame about that behavior, or they think that part is contributing to weight gain. Similarly, you may have a restricting part who other parts don't like. They might see it as being too rigid, too depriving, or just downright boring.

Some parts are on opposite sides of the fence. We say that these parts are polarized with each other, as they seem to be polar opposites. Polarized parts tend to want two different things. A great example of this is bingeing and restricting parts. As you just read, bingeing parts tend to be parts who are tired of feeling deprived and who want to use food to numb your system. Restricting parts want you to feel in control of food and may have concerns about your weight.

It's important to notice which parts are polarized with each other. These parts not only have opposite agendas, but may also have serious concerns about the other one taking over. For example, your restricting parts are very worried about your binge eating parts running the show because they want order and control with food or they're concerned that bingeing will lead to weight gain, or both. On the opposite side, binge eating parts are concerned about restrictive parts taking over because they want to be able to use food for emotional reasons or they really enjoy food and don't want to be restricted.

As a therapist, I'm always curious about who's on the other side of the fence. If a client comes in wanting to stop binge eating, I'm curious about the parts who *don't* want this to happen because they'll do what they can to ensure that it doesn't. Similarly, if a client comes in wanting to stop dieting, I'm curious about those parts *and* the ones who are terrified to stop dieting.

Recognizing that there are likely parts on the other side of the fence is incredibly important. Both parts will do their best to take over and run the show. They'll keep you locked in a constant game of ping-pong, going back and forth from one extreme to the other. This experience probably resonates with you.

How Parts Interact

The examples that follow each demonstrate interaction between an exile and a protector. These scenarios are not intended to suggest that you have the parts described in them (although you may) but are just to demonstrate what parts are and how they relate to one another.

- You've had a stressful day at work and stop at your favorite bakery for a cupcake (or two) on your way home.
  - Your exiled part doesn't feel good enough due to negative feedback at work.

- Your protector part hopes to make the exile feel better by giving it something it loves: cupcakes.

- You're at a party and someone makes a so-called joke about your appearance. You head to the bowl of chips and start munching away.
  - Your exiled part feels ashamed of your appearance.
  - Your protector part wants to push all that shame away so you can stay at the party without bursting into tears, so it heads for the chips.

- You eat an entire pint of ice cream after getting into a fight with your partner.
  - Your exiled part fears loss and abandonment.
  - Your protector part fears the exile will take over so it stuffs the fear down and numbs your system with ice cream.

- Once again, your mom tells you that she thinks you've gained too much weight, so you break out the keto cookbook and vow to start dieting tomorrow.
  - Your exiled part feels rejected and unloved by your mom.
  - Your protector part believes if you just lost weight, your mom would love and accept you, and therefore starts dieting.

I hope these examples show that your feelings, thoughts, and behaviors are all carried and caused by different parts. Eating and restricting very often start with an exiled part who becomes triggered and sets your protectors in motion to push those feelings down or soothe that exile. This explains why merely changing your eating habits has never worked. *It's never been about the behavior itself.* It's about getting to the exile underneath.

I will tell you that these examples are a bit simplistic. Very often, there are more parts involved in the process, but we'll get to that later. At this point, all I want you to know is that you have parts and to understand how they drive your eating behaviors.

How IFS Helps You Change Your Eating

Let's summarize what we've learned so far:

- We all have parts.

- We all have a Self.

- We have two different types of parts: exiles and protectors.

- Our protectors are either managers or firefighters, and their role is to protect our exiles.

At this point, you might be saying, "Okay, Kim, I think I get this whole parts thing, but what do I do with them? Do I just tell them to stop? Do I try to get rid of them? And what's the deal with this Self of mine? What do I do with that?"

All wonderful questions! Let's talk about where we go from here and what we're aiming for. There are three goals that we'll be working toward in the next couple of chapters, and all of them will help you change your relationship with food and your body for good. We'll go into more detail in subsequent chapters, but let's just get an overview now.

Getting to know your Self. It's vitally important that you connect with your Self and know when you're in Self. The Self is a huge resource for your parts, and you need to embody Self-energy when you get to know your parts. Being in Self also allows us to be Self-led in our eating and in life in general. We'll talk about what it means to be Self-led later in the book.

Getting to know the parts in your eating system. Remember that our parts are the ones who carry our thoughts and feelings and direct our behavior. Because of this, we need to get to know them *directly*. And we do this by talking to them and asking them about their experiences, jobs, beliefs, emotions, and so on. I know that may sound a little strange. I'm inviting you to talk to yourself. My guess is, if you're really being honest, you already do this. I know I do! I'm just giving you permission to do it deliberately.

Learning how to unblend from your parts. Remember what we said about blending? When our parts have grabbed the wheel and taken over, they're blended with us. We want to get some space from them—this is called unblending. Unblending is one of the most invaluable skills IFS has to offer, in my opinion. Getting space between your Self and your parts allows you to not get taken over by them. By unblending, your part can continue to feel what it's feeling without your Self feeling that emotion (or at least feeling a whole lot less of it). It also allows you not to engage in the behavior the part wants to engage in. When we unblend from our parts, we can then have a conversation with them to understand what's going on for them at that moment.

Here's another way of thinking about unblending. Imagine you and I are sitting in a therapy session. I am the Self and you are a part. There's space between us. You may become extremely emotional, but I don't. I stay calm and curious so that I can be helpful. If I take on the emotion you're experiencing, I can no longer be helpful. I'm in it with you, which means I no longer have the resources to help you.

This is what we're going for with our parts. Space. Your Self can be a resource to your parts *when you have space from them.* Believe it or not, our parts do understand this, and they will step back when you ask them to, once they understand that it's in their best interest.

Let's look at an example. Let's say you have a part who's led you to the fridge, and you're standing there grabbing all the food you can hold. That's not *you* (and by "you" I mean your Self). That's *one part* of you. And if you get space from that part, you can put down the food and have a conversation with that part. You can understand what's going on for it right now, and you can offer to help. (We'll talk about what that "help" looks like in later chapters.) Yes, you may still end up eating, but I'd be willing to bet that you'll be eating much more calmly because you've unblended from this part.

Accomplishing these goals will help you achieve your ultimate goal of Self-led eating. More to come in the final chapter, but for now, just know that when we're Self-led toward food, we're able to approach food with calmness and flexibility. Our parts are no longer running the show, making decisions that may not work well for us. When we're Self-led, we can tune into our bodies and use the skills of IE to make nourishing choices. I promise all of that will make more sense as we go along!

Common Parts

Now we're going to start looking at some common parts who seem to be in many people's eating systems (especially if those people struggle with eating concerns). When we talk about parts, what we're actually talking about is their role or behavior. For example, when I talk about a binge eating part, what I actually mean is a part who is using the behavior of binge eating to serve a certain purpose. But describing parts in that way can be quite a mouthful! In order to keep it easier to read, I'll be using titles like binge eating part or comfort eating part.

Please note that *everyone's system is different.* You may have all the parts you'll read about in this chapter, or you may have only a few. And that's okay! Whoever is in your system is allowed to be there. As we say in IFS, "All parts are welcome." There are no right or wrong parts, and there is no right or wrong system. If you read about a part and that part doesn't resonate with you, that's okay. You just may not have a part with the role I'm describing. Or you may not have noticed it before.

Protectors

Let's look at different types of protector eating parts. As you go, check the ones that you immediately resonate with. Spend a moment reflecting on that part, and then write about what you notice. Do you know what that part feels like? When it shows up? What its intentions might be?

The Comfort Eater. The comfort eater turns to food to comfort an exiled part. Some of these parts also use food to comfort or soothe themselves. Many of us have more than one comfort eating part, and many of these parts have been using food in this way for a long time. As children, food is one of the few things we can access to soothe ourselves, so this can become a pattern very early on.

☐ I have this part.

What I notice about it: _____

_____

The Binge Eater. These parts tend to be firefighters. Their job is to numb the entire system. Binge eating parts jump in when an exiled part who's carrying heavy emotions (like shame) gets triggered or activated. The binge eater is afraid that this exiled part will take over the system and flood you with shame and therefore eats in order to put you in a food coma. Binge eating parts can also jump in in reaction to restricting parts. The binge eating part may get tired of restricting and feeling deprived and therefore lead you to food in a big way.

☐ I have this part.

What I notice about it: _____

_____

The Dieter/Restrictor. You likely have more than one restrictive part, as these parts tend to have a few different roles. One role may be to restrict food in order to lose weight so that you will feel valued and accepted in our current culture. Another role may be to restrict food in order to feel a sense of control. This is a pattern that can start during childhood as well, as one of the few things kids have control over is what they put in their mouths. Finally, restrictive parts often feel very proud of their ability to eat less than others. Essentially, they're protecting parts who don't feel good enough by doing something others can't: not eating. These parts tend to think they're helping you feel special or unique.

☐ I have this part.

What I notice about it: _____

_____

The Rebel. The rebel is the part of us who's sick and tired of food restriction. This part will rebel against diet culture and/or someone in particular who has forced you to restrict your food (perhaps a parent). It will also rebel against your own parts who restrict food.

☐ I have this part.

What I notice about it: _____

_____

The Distractor. The distractor leads us to food in order to distract our parts from the exiles who are carrying painful emotions. These parts tend to believe we can't handle these emotions so they try to ensure that we don't have to, and they do this by distracting us with food.

☐ I have this part.

What I notice about it: _____

_____

The Critic. Everyone has critical parts, and they can be really hard on us about anything. Within eating systems, there can be parts who are critical about how other parts eat (for example, they eat the wrong foods, they can't stick to a diet, they binge) and about the body. And believe it or not, they're doing that to be helpful. They truly believe that if they're critical, other parts will work harder to be better, however that's defined. It's a tough-love approach that they've often learned from others.

☐ I have this part.

What I notice about it: _____

_____

The Punisher. Some of us have parts who punish other parts of our body with food. For example, if a part of you hates your body, it may actually punish it by eating so much that it feels uncomfortable. Or a part who turns to food may punish a restricting part (because it's so tired of being deprived) by eating so much that you feel sick. In my experience, not everyone has punishing parts, so you may not notice these.

☐ I have this part.

What I notice about it: _____

_____

The Blocker. This part blocks your connection to your body. It can develop for many reasons, the first being trauma. If you've had trauma inflicted on or about your physical self, it can feel very unsafe to be in your body. In order to distract or numb those uncomfortable feelings, parts can just block you from experiencing them. Additionally, if parts don't like or trust your body, they may block you from physically experiencing it. You may also have parts who don't want you to notice that you're hungry (because they don't want you to eat), so they just tune out those cues. Similarly, you may have parts who want to keep eating past the point of fullness so they block you from noticing your fullness cues. Getting to know your blocker parts is essential to implementing IE. As you read in chapter 1, the main goal of IE is attunement—connecting with your body so you can recognize what it needs. This process is incredibly difficult when parts are standing in the way.

☐ I have this part.

What I notice about it: _____

_____

The Doer. Many of us have doer parts or busy parts who keep us going, going, going nonstop, and they typically do this for a couple of reasons. First of all, these parts tend to be associated with achievement and success and believe that if we just accomplish something or reach certain goals then we're valuable and worthwhile. These parts are also really good distracting parts—if I'm going nonstop, I don't have time to focus on things I may actually be unhappy about or fearful of.

☐ I have this part.

What I notice about it: _____

_____

Thinking Parts. As you begin to get to know your parts, you may notice some thinking parts. These parts love to figure out what's going on and get to know other parts on an intellectual level. While we can appreciate their interest, they often get in the way of your Self connecting to the part you really need to connect to, so be on the lookout for those thinkers!

☐ I have this part.

What I notice about it: _____

_____

Therapist Parts. If you happen to be a therapist, it's very likely that your highly trained clinician parts will also be present during the process of getting to know other parts. Like the thinkers, these parts tend to be *very* curious about what's going on because these discussions are right up their alley. They may want to impose their clinical opinion on the process, so be on the lookout for them also!

☐ I have this part.

What I notice about it: _____

_____

As you can see, there are many possible protective parts in your eating system. What other parts are you noticing now that you're thinking about it? Note them here:

_____

_____

_____

_____

_____

_____

_____

Exiles

Now that we've looked at the parts who protect, let's look at the exiled parts who are being protected. Remember that our exiles carry extreme emotions and beliefs that have resulted from trauma and other negative experiences. I recognize that these parts may be hard to face because of what they're carrying, but you don't have to take a deep dive into them right now. This is just a time to notice what exiles tend to carry and for you to understand that these are the parts who are underneath your protective parts.

Let's look a little more closely at these exiles, starting with parts who carry shame.

Shame Parts. Shame is a very painful emotion that our parts don't want to feel. It results from the belief that you are flawed, wrong, or bad. Very often, we have strong protectors that make sure we don't feel shame. They may be the ones noted above, but they don't have to be. Parts that protect shame don't have to use food to do so, but they certainly can. Many of us have more than one shame part. And these parts carry shame about different aspects of ourselves. You may have a part who feels shame about your body, another part who carries shame about your out-of-control eating, and another part who feels shame about your finances. These are likely all different parts.

☐ I have this part.

What I notice about it: _____

_____

Not-Good-Enough Parts. Similarly, many of us have parts who don't feel good enough or believe that they aren't lovable. Again, different parts carry these feelings about different aspects of ourselves. You may have a part who feels your body isn't good enough, another part who feels the degree you've earned isn't good enough, and another part who thinks your house is too small. Other parts may point to qualities that support their belief that you're unlovable.

☐ I have this part.

What I notice about it: _____

_____

Loneliness. Many, if not most, of us have parts who carry feelings of loneliness. We've probably all had times in our lives when we felt disconnected from others, and it's easy to see how exiles can pick up the burden of loneliness. Also, as you already read, many of our parts don't know our Self, and they may know few, if any, other parts. This can also lead to loneliness.

☐   I have this part.

What I notice about it: _____

_____

I'm Too Sensitive/Too Much. Many of us have been told during our lives that we're "too much" or "too sensitive," and we may therefore have parts who still carry those beliefs. When these parts take over, you may feel shame about having emotions. Your system may work really hard to keep you quiet and small because taking up space feels dangerous. You may also have difficulty asking for what you need because these parts believe that you're asking for too much or don't deserve to even have needs.

☐   I have this part.

What I notice about it: _____

_____

Again, this is not an exhaustive list of the potential parts within an eating system, and it may not accurately reflect your own system. We're all different, and so are our parts. I hope you're now thinking about and noticing your own parts. We'll be getting to know them much more fully in the coming chapters. For now, however, I suggest spending time with the questions that follow, prompting you to notice the parts within this chapter that resonate with you.

Checking In

In order to deepen your understanding and awareness of your parts, take the time to reflect on and respond to these questions.

What parts from the list seem to resonate the most with you?

_____

_____

_____

How do these parts resonate? Where are they in your body? What are they saying?

_____

_____

_____

_____

What parts seem difficult for you to accept or connect with?

_____

_____

_____

What parts do you feel you already know fairly well?

_____

_____

_____

CHAPTER 3

Getting to Know Your Self

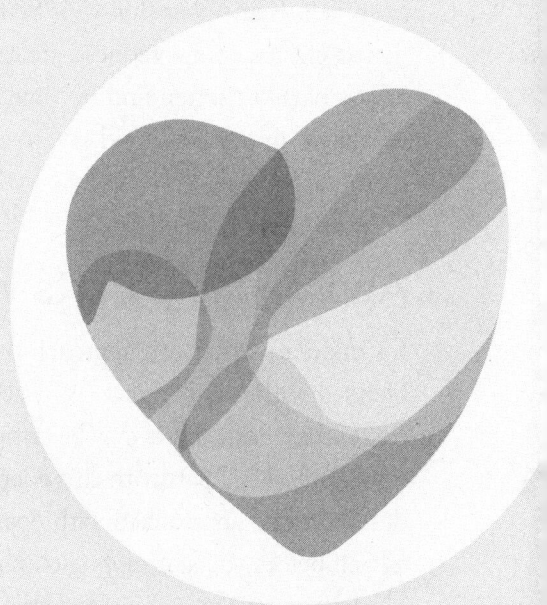

Now that you have learned about how IFS works, it's time to get a better understanding of your Self. We're all composed of many different parts and a core Self. And it's vitally important that you learn what it's like to be in Self, or to embody Self-energy, because we *always* want to approach our parts from Self. Remember that your Self is composed of the 8 C's: compassion, curiosity, calmness, confidence, clarity, connectedness, creativity, and courage. Self approaches *all* parts with this energy, which allows parts to soften and become less extreme. Self-energy heals our parts and allows them to feel validated, understood, and safe to shift their roles.

Approaching Parts with Self-Energy

It's imperative that we approach our parts with our Self-energy instead of approaching them while blended with another part. Why? Because our parts aren't always curious and compassionate toward each other. Some parts may be critical or feel negative toward the part we're trying to get to know and if we approach a part with this energy, it may retreat, feel shame, or rebel and act out. All of our parts deserve to be approached with open, curious Self-energy, and you *must* be able to know when you're in Self before you start approaching your parts.

Let me give you an example that demonstrates the difference between approaching one part while blended with another versus approaching a part with Self-energy. Let's say you have a binge eating part you'd like to get to know and you have a restrictive part who's polarized with it and doesn't like that it's bingeing. Here's what it might look like if you approach your binge eating part while you're blended with the restrictive part:

You: Hey, why do you keep bingeing? Don't you see how much I hate that?

Binge Eating Part: Well, I actually think what I do is helpful.

You: Helpful? Are you kidding me? What you're doing is terrible! How could it be helpful?

Binge Eating Part: It just is. It helps us deal with things.

You: That doesn't make any sense!

Binge Eating Part: (Crickets—the part has stopped communicating)

In this example, all the negative energy coming from the restrictive part has shut down the binge eating part. The binge eating part may also have become defensive or possibly headed straight back to food in rebellion.

Now let's look at a possible conversation with the binge eating part when we approach it with Self-energy:

You (Self): I would really like to get to know you, binge eating part. Please share with me whatever you'd like me to know about you.

Binge Eating Part: Really? No one has ever wanted to get to know me before.

You: I get that. I think some of my other parts don't like what you're doing—but they don't understand what you're doing. I'd really like to understand you because I know you're just trying to help me.

Binge Eating Part: Yes! All I've ever wanted to do is help! No one sees that.

You: I do! And I'd love to help you too. Can you tell me more about you?

Can you see how different that energy is? The binge eating part immediately feels heard and supported. This opens up a conversation with the part. This is why we must be in Self when we get to know our parts.

Chances are, you've experienced being in Self before, but you didn't realize it or didn't have a name for it. Try to recall a time when you felt calm, curious, and compassionate. Or maybe a time when you felt really connected to another person, or perhaps very confident in yourself. Describe that experience and tell what it felt like.

_____

_____

_____

_____

_____

_____

_____

_____

_____

For some people, being in nature automatically brings about Self-energy. Just being present under the sun or the stars, feeling the breeze on your face, or enjoying the beautiful colors of a forest or sunset can easily bring out our calmness and compassion. Similarly, if you're someone who enjoys being creative, you are likely in Self during those moments. There is often no agenda at those times— just you channeling your creativity and allowing it to go wherever it would like. That's Self-energy.

We are often able to bring Self-energy toward others more easily than we are toward ourselves. Think about how you feel toward the significant people in your life. Most likely, you've had moments of feeling very compassionate toward and curious about them. You have no agenda toward them—you just love them. That's what Self-energy feels like.

Take a moment to think about someone who you love deeply and unconditionally. How are you feeling when you think about them? Write about how that open, compassionate energy feels.

_____

_____

_____

_____

_____

_____

_____

_____

How Do You Know If You're in Self?

When our Self-energy is present, we tend to feel calm, open, and curious. We're able to offer others and ourselves compassion, and we don't have an agenda about anything. We feel connected to our parts and to those around us. We aren't judgmental, we aren't trying to control anything or anyone, and we aren't rattled by anything.

Imagine approaching food in this way. When you approach food and eating with Self-energy instead of through your parts, you can notice your hunger levels and what you're hungry for. You can tune into your body, recognize what it needs, and do your best to provide for it. Foods that have been "fear" foods or "forbidden" foods are approached with calmness because they don't have the same draw to your Self as they do to your parts. And finally, you can check in with the parts of you that lead you to food and offer them what they really need, which often isn't food.

Similarly, when you approach your body with Self-energy, you're no longer focused on its appearance and its size. Self *does not care about your weight.* That may seem very hard to believe, but it's true. When you approach your body with Self-energy, you *want* to treat it with the respect it deserves, and you do your best to nourish it with whatever it needs. You also notice what movement and activities it enjoys and engage in them when you're able to.

You may already be resonating with this idea of Self-energy and know that you've experienced it before. Or you may be saying "But Kim, I hate nature, I can't draw stick figures, and I tend to be pretty critical of myself!" That's okay! I promise you that there's a Self in there. Remember that you don't need to have access to all 8 C qualities in order to be in Self. Even having a good amount of one is enough.

Noticing Your Self-Energy

Let's connect to your Self-energy with meditation. Feel free to read this meditation to yourself or visit http://www.newharbinger.com/57286 to download an audio version. Before you begin this process, be sure that you'll have at least fifteen minutes of quiet time to yourself in order to really get into the exercise. And be sure that the space you're in feels calm and that your body is in a comfortable position. You may want to turn on some soft music, grab a fuzzy blanket, or light a candle.

Begin by softening your gaze or closing your eyes, whichever feels comfortable to your system. Take a deep breath in and then slowly exhale. Turn your attention inward. Continue focusing on your breathing and notice how your body feels with each inhale and exhale. Feel your shoulders drop, your breathing slow.

When you are ready, imagine a place that feels safe and comfortable, that's beautiful and peaceful. Notice the colors in this place. The sounds. The smells. And notice the connection you feel to this place. Maybe it's a place you've already been to. Or it may be a place you've only dreamed of. Notice the feeling of calm and clarity while you're in this space. Continue your breathing, in and out, and with every out-breath, visualize your calm, connected, compassionate, confident Self-energy filling this beautiful space.

It may be helpful to see your Self-energy as a beautiful light emanating from you. Or it may look like a calm river flowing by. Just notice this wonderful energy that emanates from you.

Now, invite any of your parts who are curious to be present with you. You may be able to see them or hear them. You may just have a felt-sense of them. Let all your parts know that they are welcome. Send all your parts your compassion. Your calmness. Your Self-energy. And notice what happens when you do. Notice how your parts are responding to you. Notice the changes in your body. Take some time to just notice.

Let your parts know that you need to get back to your life now, but that you're a resource for them. Let them know that you're very curious about all of them and hope to meet them soon. Invite them to stay in this calm, beautiful space for as long as they would like. And when you're ready, open your eyes and return to your space.

How did it go? Take a moment to reflect on your experience by answering these questions:

What did you notice when you tried to access your Self-energy? What happened?

_____

_____

_____

_____

_____

Were you able to access your Self-energy? If so, how could you tell?

_____

_____

_____

_____

What C quality did you notice the most when you were in Self?

_____

_____

_____

What other C qualities, if any, did you notice?

_____

_____

_____

If this exercise felt strange to you or if you feel like it didn't work, that's okay. Noticing your Self-energy may be new and different for you, and it takes practice. Also, very often, we have parts who are trying so hard to get it right that they block our Self-energy. Or you may have parts who think this is weird and will also obstruct the process. Please be patient with those parts. They're just trying to protect you.

I recommend repeating this meditation on a regular basis in order to strengthen your ability to access your Self-energy quickly and easily. The more you practice, the easier it gets. Set aside time on a daily basis if possible (if that's too much, do what works for you) and keep practicing—you'll get there.

I also recommend continuing to practice accessing your Self-energy before moving ahead in this book. Again, we *must* approach our parts with Self-energy. If you're not there yet, that's okay—take your time and keep practicing. The last thing you want to do is move forward before you're ready.

CHAPTER 4

Getting to Know Your Protector Parts

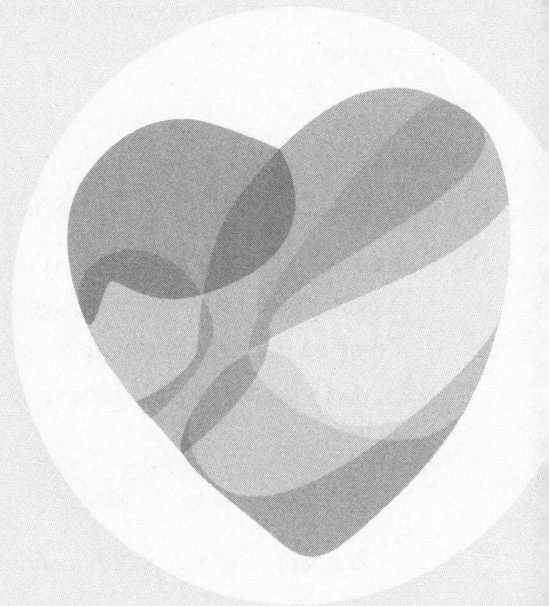

In chapter 3, you learned how to access your Self-energy. If you need to spend more time learning to recognize and find Self-energy, please do so before moving on. But, if you now know what it feels like to have Self-energy, you can start getting to know your parts. First, we'll work on the process of identifying your parts and mapping your system. Then, we'll dig deeper into getting to know your protector parts.

Discovering Parts by Noticing Your Thoughts

Your thoughts are essentially your parts speaking to you, so when you notice your thoughts, you're noticing your parts. Every thought you have is a part talking to you. When you have a lot of thoughts, it may be the same part with a lot to say, or you may have many parts chiming in.

Let's consider this example. If I were to pause and record my thoughts right now, they would include:

It feels so nice to be sitting by the fire right now.

Yes, but it's smoky and that annoys me.

I'm kind of getting tired sitting here—I don't move enough.

I kind of want a snack.

You don't need a snack—you're not hungry.

Let's just get back to writing.

I know that isn't very exciting dialogue, but each one of those sentences is another part talking. Each thought is a different part who's noticing or wanting something different or is having a different experience than the others.

It's your turn to give it a shot. Here's how:

- Find a quiet space and grab something to write with.

- Get comfy and take some deep breaths.

- Notice what thoughts come into your mind. These are your parts.

- Spend some time noticing what they're saying. Try to notice as many as you can.

- Offer your parts Self-energy, and thank them for being with you.

Jot down all the thoughts you just noticed.

_____

_____

_____

_____

_____

Noticing your thoughts can help you identify parts who play different roles in your experience with food as well. For example, I have parts who enjoy having a snack at night. If I were to stop to notice the thoughts that come up as I begin thinking about a snack, they might sound something like this:

I want a snack.

Wait—I don't need a snack.

Here she goes again—she has no self-control.

You can't eat another snack—you'll gain weight.

Geez—it's just one snack—what's the big deal?

Do you see how there are different parts talking here? A part who wants a snack, one who doesn't, one who's concerned about weight, one who feels out of control, and one who's trying to figure out what all the fuss is about.

Go ahead and imagine a recent time when you engaged in a behavior surrounding food, such as emotional eating, binge eating, or restricting. Notice the thoughts that come up and jot them down.

_____

_____

_____

_____

_____

As I hope you're starting to realize, we tend to have quite a few parts who have strong thoughts and feelings about food. One part suggesting an evening snack can lead to a whole crew of parts with different thoughts and feelings about that *one* snack. *This is why changing eating patterns is so difficult.* We tend to view eating as just a habit or a behavior that we need to change, but it's much more complicated than that.

Let's take some time to reflect on the experience of noticing your thoughts (parts) by answering these questions.

How was it for you to notice your thoughts?

_____

_____

_____

_____

Were you able to recognize your thoughts as parts? What, if anything, was difficult about that?

_____

_____

_____

_____

Were there any thoughts (parts) that surprised you?

_____

_____

_____

_____

Mapping Your Eating System

Now that you have an idea of what it's like to tune in and notice your parts, it's time to find parts within your eating system. We're going to create a map of your system so that you have a much clearer idea of all the parts who contribute to your relationship with food and your body. I don't remotely expect you to notice all the parts in your eating system right now. Consider this to be a living document that you will likely be contributing to for some time. It may never be quite finished, and that's okay! But it will be helpful to begin noticing who's in there.

A parts map is essentially what it sounds like—a map of your internal system. There are a few different ways to map your system, and we'll start with a simple one: listing your parts.

Go back to chapter 2 and review the list of common parts. Now, add the parts you thought were in your eating system to the list on the following page. Then, go back to the end of chapter 1, where I asked you what fears and concerns you have about getting started with IFS and IE. Those are parts as well, and they belong on the map. If you run out of space on the list that follows, or if you'd like to print out another list, head to http://www.newharbinger.com/57286 for blank copies.

My Parts List

_____

_____

_____

_____

_____

_____

_____

_____

_____

_____

_____

_____

_____

_____

_____

_____

_____

_____

Now, take some time to answer the questions below to notice even more parts. Add every part you notice to your parts list and indicate if the part seems like a protector or an exile. (Remember, protectors tend to engage in behaviors, exiles tend to carry emotions.)

What are the behaviors surrounding food that you have concerns about or would like to change?

_____

_____

_____

_____

_____

_____

What other behaviors do you engage in around food? List everything you can think of from binge eating to meal prep to dieting.

_____

_____

_____

_____

_____

_____

What beliefs or rules do you tend to carry about food? These may include needing to abstain from certain foods, believing that food is either healthy or unhealthy, or needing to limit calories.

_____

_____

_____

_____

_____

_____

What feelings and beliefs do you have about your body? How do you talk to yourself about your body?

_____

_____

_____

_____

_____

_____

_____

By this point, you likely have a good-sized list of parts. That's great! You can move forward to getting to know your parts with this list, or, if you're more visual, you can draw a map of your parts. This gives you a visual of your system, which for some folx is really helpful. You can draw your parts in different sizes and colors, and you can place them near or far from each other.

Here's an example of what a parts map may look like for someone who has an emotional eating part (that's the part in the center). In it, you can see that the parts are different sizes and are placed in different relationships to each other. I've also indicated if the part is likely a protector or an exile.

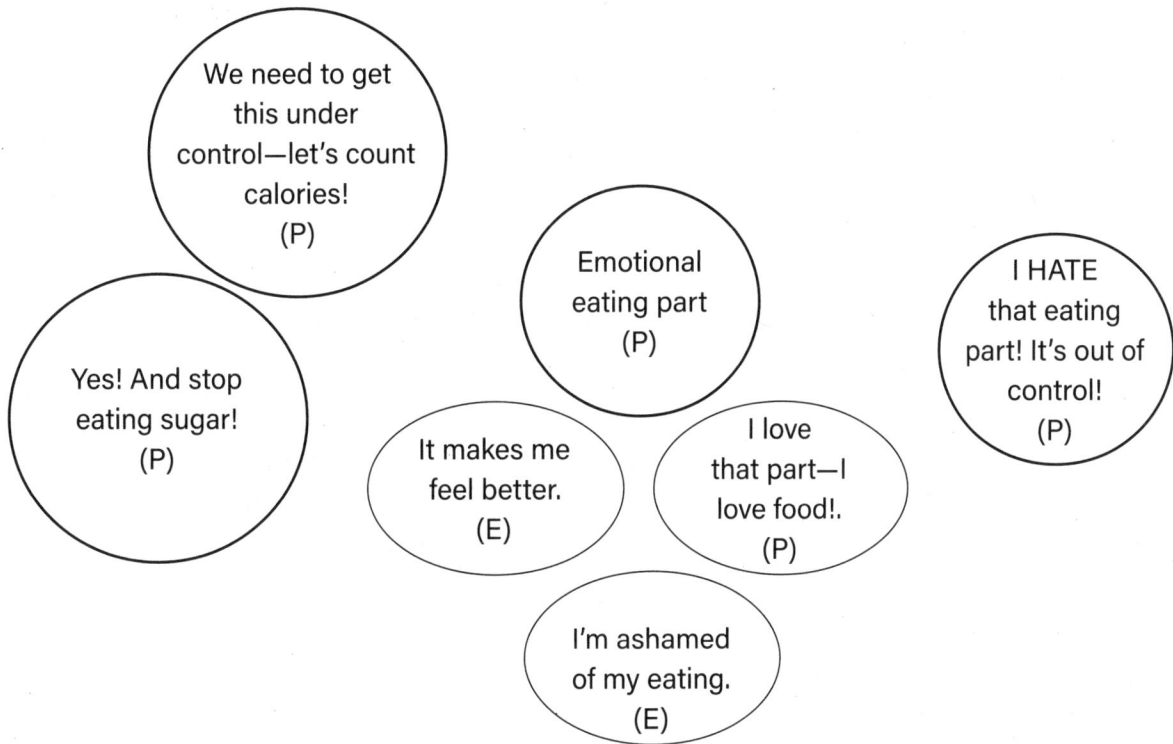

We need to get this under control—let's count calories! (P)

Yes! And stop eating sugar! (P)

Emotional eating part (P)

I HATE that eating part! It's out of control! (P)

It makes me feel better. (E)

I love that part—I love food!. (P)

I'm ashamed of my eating. (E)

Now it's your turn. Visit http://www.newharbinger.com/57286 for blank copies of this map to print out, or create your own, using the map on the following page. Look at your list of parts and choose one that you're curious about and that has some significance in your system. Put that part in the middle of the map, and think about what other parts might relate or react to this part. Place these parts around the original part, however they seem to fit. This is *your* parts map!

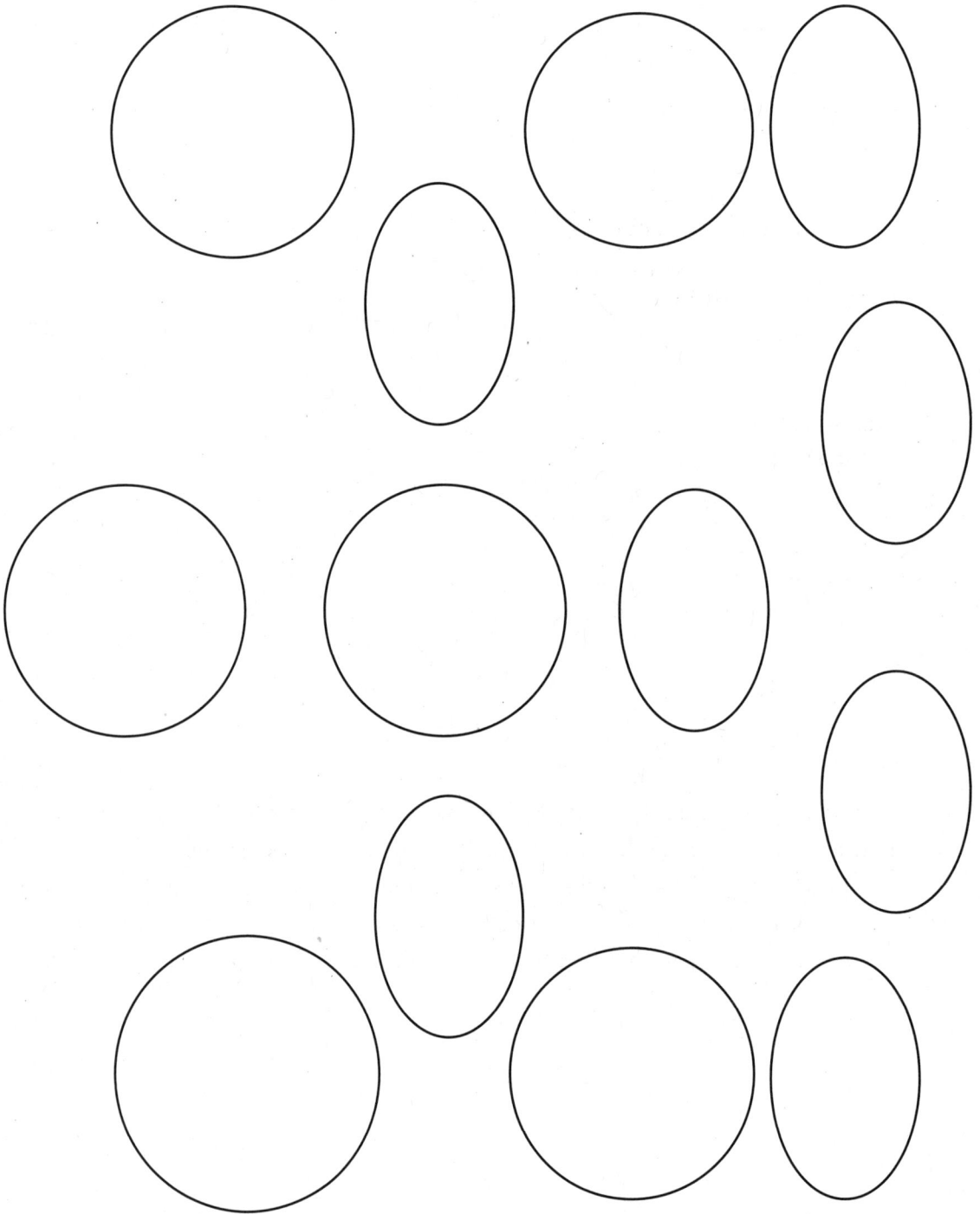

My Parts Map

The third way to map out parts is to draw each one separately. Picture the part in your mind's eye, and start drawing, using blank paper or a journal. You can even use AI to create images of your parts. Remember, everyone's parts look different, so start your drawing with an open mind. Once you've drawn your parts, you can lay them out on a surface and place them however they seem to relate to each other.

Getting to Know Your Protectors

Now that you've learned how to notice and map your parts, let's take things a step further and really get to *know* them. We'll start with our protectors. Exiles can overwhelm your system with emotion, and we obviously don't want that to happen. Our protectors don't tend to like it when we go straight to an exile. They protect them for a reason, and if we bypass the protector, they won't trust us to try this again. And finally, working with exiles takes a different skill set that we'll be getting to in chapter 5.

The distinction between a protector and an exile isn't always clear until you start talking to them, but in general, protectors are the ones engaging in an actual behavior. In contrast, parts who have feelings or beliefs (like believing you aren't good enough, that your body isn't good enough, or feeling shame or sadness) are more likely to be exiles. To review the typical parts and notice the differences between protectors and exiles, look back at chapter 2.

Before starting this practice, read through its steps. Choose a time when you'll have at least thirty minutes to yourself. Find a comfortable place and position for your body, and try to limit distractions. Some people like to put their hand on their heart doing this practice, as it seems to connect them more to their Self-energy. It's often helpful to do this with your eyes closed so that you can truly tune into your internal world; if that's not comfortable for you, just soften your gaze.

Step 1: Choose a target part. When we get to know parts, we focus on one part at a time. We call that part our target part. We choose only one part so that we can give it our full and undivided attention, allowing us to truly understand it and ensuring that it will know we're there.

You can select a part from your parts list or map or by noticing what part seems to need your attention in the moment. I suggest starting with a manager instead of a firefighter. Firefighters can be more intense than managers, and you might want to have a little more practice before getting to know them.

Step 2: Find the part. Start the process by finding the target part in or around your body. Our parts tend to get our attention with physical sensations, so just notice what your body is telling you. It may be outside your body as well. It may seem like it's across the room from you—that's okay too.

Step 3: Embody Self-energy. Once you've found the part, notice how you're feeling toward it. If you're feeling anything other than Self-energy (that is, open, curious, compassionate), you're blended with a part. For example, if you're feeling nervous, that's a part. If you hear yourself saying "I don't like that part," or "I'm frustrated toward it," those are parts. Remember that we *always* want to approach our parts with Self-energy, so if you're feeling anything other than Self-energy, ask that part(s) to step or settle back. After you ask this part or parts to step back, check in again to see how you're feeling toward the target part. Again, if it's anything other than Self-energy, ask that part or parts to step back. Continue asking parts to step back until just Self is present. When you put your attention on the target part, you should be feeling mostly Self-energy toward it.

Not all parts will settle back when you ask them to. That's a normal part of the process. These parts either have something they really want you to know, or they're concerned about you getting to know the target part. They may be afraid that if you talk to the target part, it will grab the wheel and never leave. Or they may fear that you're trying to get rid of the part. Many times, giving the parts some reassurance that you won't let the target part take over or that you aren't trying to get rid of it is all your parts need to allow them to settle back.

If a part just won't step back, then we make *it* our new target part, and we go through the process of getting to know that part. That means you start from the beginning by finding the part in or around your body and noticing how you feel toward it. Once you have Self-energy toward that part, proceed with the next step.

Step 4: Befriend the part. Now that you've noticed the part, are aware of how you're experiencing it, and know that you have Self-energy toward it, it's time to get to know the part better, and it's time for the part to get to know you. When you get to know a protector, you're gaining some answers:

- Do they know who you are? You want to be sure that your parts know who Self is before proceeding so that they know they have a resource, a partner, a colleague. If the part doesn't know who you are, let it know that you're the grown-up version of the part, that it's a part of you. Let it know that you value it and all your parts, and you're here to get to know it better.

- How old are they? Very often, parts will tell you their exact age. Sometimes, they aren't really sure. That's all fine.

- Does it know how old you are? If the part doesn't know or thinks you're an age other than your actual age, give it an update and notice how it responds to this information.

- What is the part's job in your system? To get very specific information, ask the part:

  - What is your job?

  - How long have you had this job?

  - What do you like about it?

  - What don't you like?

- What is it afraid will happen if it no longer does its job? This is the question that can lead us to an exile. When a part answers this question, it often says things like, "I'm afraid I'll gain so much weight that no one will want me." Or "I'm afraid I'll just be overwhelmed." Or "I'm afraid I'll be really sad." These are indications that this part is protecting an exile who feels body shame, feels overwhelmed, or is carrying sadness (respectively).

In the next chapter, you'll learn how to proceed if this part leads you to an exile. For now, just place the exile on your parts map.

Step 5: Ask how you can help. Now that you've gotten to know this part, it's time to see what it needs from you. Ask the part how you can be helpful to it. (This is a wonderful question to ask all your parts. You can hear directly from them what they'd like from you, if they even know. They may not. If they didn't know there was a Self, they may have a hard time coming up with a way for you to help them.)

Here are some possible responses a part may have:

- The part may say that it's exhausted and wants a break, but it feels like it can't stop. If that's the case, you can offer to help the part do its job. Ask the part to give you a signal when it needs your help, or let it know you'll be on the lookout for it and will offer help when you notice it stepping in.

- The part may really want to drop its job but may be afraid that no one else will do it. In that case, let it know that you can be helpful. Spend some time with the part discussing what aspects of the job it's willing to let you try, even if just briefly. You can then make the commitment to check back in later to see how it's going and whether the part would like to hand over more of the job to you.

- The part may just want to hang out with you for a bit. If you're able to in the moment, go ahead and spend time with the part. If you can't, make a commitment to come back at a later time to spend time with it. Ask it where it would like to hang out until then. This place can be real, like in your living room or at the beach, or imaginary.

Step 6: Check in and offer gratitude. Now that you're wrapping things up with this part, it's time to offer your thanks and ask the part how often it would like you to check in.

- When we get to know our parts, we want to continue the connection. Make a commitment to talking to the part at another time, preferably within the next day or two. The more present you are for the part, the more it will begin to trust you, and the more it will allow you to be helpful.

- Thank the part for all it does for you. This is yet another incredibly important piece. Our parts are generally not used to being thanked by us. The parts who use food in various ways are used to being vilified and told to stop what they're doing. Receiving a Self-led, heartfelt thank-you from you speaks volumes to your parts. Not all parts will trust that in the beginning or will be able to accept it, but just keep sending thanks to your parts.

- Check in with any parts who you met and unblended from at the beginning of this process. Ask them what they noticed about the part you got to know and if there's anything they need from you. If there is, do your best to provide it.

I know it can seem like a lot of information to ask a part. It's completely understandable to feel confused or overwhelmed right now. But the more you practice the process, the easier it gets. And again, you have meditations available to you to walk you through it.

I also want you to know that when you're going through this process, you don't want to just ask these questions rapid-fire. You don't have to go in a specific order. You want this to be a conversation between your Self and the part, so just take it as it flows. Let your curiosity guide the process. Notice if you're asking questions from your heart or from your head. If they seem to be coming from your head, you aren't in Self. Take a moment to ask your curious, thinking parts to step back and give your Self the space to connect with this part.

Your Turn: Getting to Know a Protector Part

Now that you understand the process, you can begin connecting with a protector part. Below, the process is spelled out with space to write in your part's responses if you so choose. At http://www. newharbinger.com/57286, you'll find a blank copy of this process to print and use as many times as you need. You can also download a recorded meditation that will guide you through the process.

Be sure you have enough time to complete the process, ideally at least thirty minutes. Find a space where you won't be distracted, and get into a comfortable position.

Step 1: Choose a target part. Look back at your parts map and notice which parts you're curious about. (Again, be sure to start with a manager). Choose up to five of these parts and list them here.

1. _____

2. _____

3. _____

4. _____

5. _____

Now, choose a part to begin with. Select a part who doesn't seem overwhelming to you and whom you have some Self-energy toward. If more than one fits the bill, just pick one. You'll be returning to the list to get to know all of your parts, so reassure them that you aren't leaving them behind.

My target part is: _____

Step 2: Find the part. Once you're comfortable, turn your attention inward. Focus on your bodily sensations, and notice where the part is, in or around your body. Remember that the part may be outside of your body.

Once you've found the part, ask yourself these questions:

How do I experience the part? Do I see it? Hear it? Feel it?

_____

_____

_____

If I see it, what does it look like? What color or shape is it? How large or small is it?

_____

_____

_____

_____

If I hear it, what is it saying?

_____

_____

_____

_____

If I feel it, what sensation am I experiencing?

_____

_____

_____

_____

If the part is outside of my body, how close is it to me? (If it seems too close, ask it to step back just a little to give you space. If it's so far away that it's hard to connect to, you can either move toward it or ask it to come closer to you.)

_____

_____

Step 3: Embody Self-energy. How do I feel toward the part? (If you're blended with another part, ask that part to step back. Once it does, place your attention on the target part and ask again. Continue this process until you know your Self is present with the target part.)

Step 4: Befriend the part. Turn your curious Self-energy toward the part and ask it:

Do you know who I am? (If not, let it know.)

_____

What would you like me to know about you?

_____

_____

_____

_____

How old are you?

_____

How old do you think I am? (If the part doesn't know or thinks you're a different age, let it know your actual age and what your life is like now.)

_____

What job do you have?

_____

_____

_____

_____

How long have you had this job?

_____

_____

How did you get this job?

_____

_____

What do you like about your job? What do you not like?

_____

_____

_____

_____

What are you afraid will happen if you no longer do your job?

_____

_____

_____

_____

What else, if anything, would you like me to know about you?

_____

_____

_____

_____

_____

_____

Step 5: Ask how you can help.

What do you need from me?

_____

_____

How can I be a resource for you?

_____

_____

Step 6: Check in and offer gratitude.

Let's think about a time for me to check in with you again. When would you like that to happen?

_____

Thank you for all you do for me. I recognize even more now how hard you've been working for me, and I want you to know how much I appreciate you.

I'd like to check in with the parts I met at the beginning of this process. What did you notice about the part we just met?

_____

_____

Is there anything you need from me?

_____

_____

Checking In

Take a few moments to reflect on what that process was like for you.

How was it for you to get to know a protector part?

_____

_____

_____

_____

_____

What did you learn from the part?

_____

_____

_____

What, if anything, was surprising about what you learned from the part?

_____

_____

_____

How are your other parts responding to this process? Are they excited? Confused? Relieved? Check inside to notice.

_____

_____

_____

You've just learned the essential crux of IFS. Yay! Connecting to, listening to, understanding, and thanking our protector parts is one of the most important pieces of IFS. Remember to check in with the parts you meet so they begin to trust your Self.

Be sure to continue getting to know your protector parts before moving on to your exiles. You definitely want to be comfortable with the process of connecting to Self-energy, unblending, and having conversations with your parts before you begin working with your exiles.

CHAPTER 5

Connecting With Your Exiles

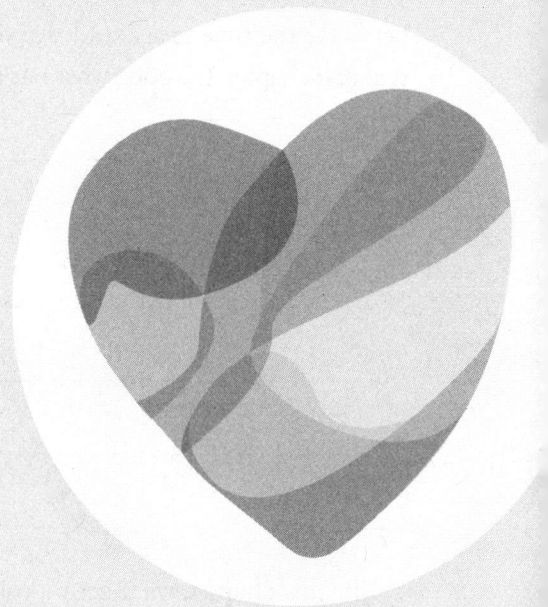

By this point, you have a much deeper understanding of who you are and how you relate to food. You've connected to your Self-energy, practiced unblending from parts, and gotten to know some of your protectors. You've accomplished so much!

Let's take the time to acknowledge your progress. Look back at the questions at the end of the introduction and chapter 1. Notice what has changed for you, and jot down your thoughts here:

_____

_____

_____

_____

_____

In this chapter, we'll get to know your exiled parts and the burdens they carry. Being seen and validated by your Self is incredibly healing for these parts. It's important to note that working with exiles can be difficult. Your exiles can easily overwhelm your system if you are unable to maintain Self-energy while connecting with them, which can lead to a lack of trust in Self by your protector parts.

I strongly recommend working with an IFS therapist or practitioner during this process if at all possible. (See the resource list at the end of the book for information on finding a therapist). An IFS therapist can help you to unburden your exiles, which means helping them to let go of the burdens they carry. The process of unburdening is beyond the scope of this book and should be done with the help of a trained professional. If you are unable to work with an IFS therapist or practitioner, you are still doing amazing work by connecting to and listening to your exiles. The process of witnessing and validating their experiences is incredibly healing on its own.

To refresh your memory, exiles are the parts of you who are carrying extreme thoughts and beliefs they picked up during a difficult or traumatic experience. I think of exiles as parts who are carrying all our heavy stuff—really painful feelings, memories from difficult experiences, and/or the beliefs we hold about ourselves that we'd rather no one else know. They tend to be young parts who are stuck in the past, and they often feel lonely and uncared for.

You might be noticing some of your own exiles right now. You may be feeling some sadness about past events or recalling difficult experiences in your life. Those feelings and memories are being held by your exiled parts, and it's completely understandable that they are making themselves known right now. You might also be noticing some compassion arising in your system right now, which is also understandable. Just thinking about these hurt parts can easily bring about your compassionate Self-energy.

Exiled parts are different from protector parts for many reasons, one being that they don't have a job in your system. They are just there, sitting with painful feelings and beliefs about themselves. Because of this, getting to know exiles is a different process than getting to know protectors, as you'll soon read.

Take a moment to notice what's happening in your system as you read more about exiles. Are you noticing your Self-energy? Are you noticing your exiles? What are you feeling in your body? Describe your experience here:

_____

_____

_____

_____

_____

Getting to Know Your Exiles

Sometimes it's very easy to know if a part is an exile. If you know it's carrying intense feelings of sadness or shame, for example, or if you know a part feels worthless, then you know it's very likely to be an exile. You may be able to look at your parts map and notice a few exiles immediately. Another way to tell is to ask the part what job it has. Exiles don't have a job in your system, so if a part answers that it has no job, you know it's an exile.

As we discussed in the previous chapter, very often we meet an exile when we ask a protector part what it's afraid will happen if it no longer does its job. For example, if you're connecting with an emotional eating part who states that it's afraid to stop eating because it's afraid you'll be too sad, you know it's protecting an exile who's carrying a lot of sadness. You would then make the exile the target part and start the process of getting to know the exile from the beginning—that is, noticing where the part is in your body, unblending from other parts, and asking what the part would like you to know about itself.

Just like we did with getting to know protectors, I'll start by describing the whole process and then provide you with an abbreviated version. It's very important that you're comfortable with this process before starting, and it's imperative that you're able to approach your exiles with Self-energy.

Step 1: Choose a target part. This process can begin in one of two ways: if you've already identified an exile you're curious about (maybe from your parts map), you can name this exile as your target part and begin the process.

However, you may have identified an exile while getting to know a protector. If this occurred, ask the protector if it's willing to introduce you to the exiled part. If a protector isn't willing to introduce you to the exile, let it know that's okay. You *never* want to push the issue. Ask the protector what it would need to feel safe allowing you to meet the exile. It may not know. It may just need some time to get to know and trust you. Be sure to respect its wishes.

Very often, protectors are willing to introduce you to an exile, but they may want to hang around to make sure things go smoothly. That's fine. At that point, make the exile your target part and start at the beginning.

Step 2: Find the part. Notice where the part is in or around your body. How are you experiencing it?

Step 3: Embody Self-energy. Now that you've found the part, notice how you're feeling toward it. If you're feeling anything other than Self-energy (curious, calm compassionate, open), those are parts. Gently ask them to give you some space. If any of them are unable to do that, make them your target part and complete the process with that part).

Step 4: Befriend the part. Engage with the part with your Self-energy.

- Ask if the part knows who you are. If it doesn't, introduce your Self as the grown-up version of the part.

- Ask the part how old it is and how old it thinks you are. If it doesn't know your correct age, update the part.

- Ask the part what it would like you to know about itself. Invite it to share whatever it feels comfortable sharing regarding its feelings and experiences. Offer it compassion, validation, and support. This can take a few minutes, or you may need to do this over a span of time. It's *very important* to take your time with this and not rush the process. It takes as long as it takes.

- Some exiles can't or would rather not use words to tell you how they feel and what happened to them. That's okay. You can ask them to show you pictures or memories of their experience. If you feel you can do this, ask it to blend just a little with you so you can feel what it's feeling. Again, you don't want the part to overwhelm you with emotion. It's almost like asking the part to hand you a little piece of its emotion so you get a flavor of what it's feeling.

- Ask the part if it's carrying any beliefs about itself, as exiles very often pick up beliefs based on their experiences. For example, maybe the exile is talking about how lonely it felt because its mom was never home. Yes, that exile is carrying immense loneliness, but it may also be carrying the belief that it's not lovable, and that's why Mom left. You can simply ask, "Did your experience lead you to take on any beliefs about yourself?"

- Once the exile has told you everything it needs you to know, ask it if it feels as if you really understand what it's saying, that you truly get it. If it says no, check in with yourself and make sure there are no other parts in the way. Be sure that you're in Self. If you are, invite it to share more.

Step 5: Ask how you can help and check in. Now that you've listened to this exiled part, ask it how you can be helpful. Be sure to validate its experiences and let it know how much you understand it.

- Many exiles just want to be heard by Self. They may tell you that they just want to be with you––let them know that you're happy to spend time with them.

- The part may also want to leave where they are and go to a place that feels safe. Ask them if they'd like to be somewhere real or imaginary. If they want to create their own safe space, help them to do that. Imagine the colors, textures, and furnishings this space would have.

- Ask how frequently the part would like you to check in with it. The IFS community recommends checking in with exiled parts daily for three weeks. If the exile wants something different, that's okay. Just be sure to ask, as it helps to build trust between your Self and your parts.

Step 6: Reconnect with the protector part. Now that you've gotten to know the exile that is being protected, it's time to return to the part who was protecting it.

Now that you've gotten to know the exile, ask the part how else you can be helpful to it and what it needs from you, if anything, at this point. It may need nothing, or it may need to just be with you. If you have time, stay with it. If it no longer needs you or you need get back to your daily life, ask where it would like to hang out (again, either real or imaginary), and allow it to go there. Ask how soon it would like you to return to it, and make a plan to do so.

- See if you can find the part who was protecting the exile you just met. Did it notice what happened with the exile? If not, let it know. If it did see what happened, ask how it feels about that.

- Ask if the protector sees its job any differently now that you've met the exile. It may not, but it may now see its job as less necessary because Self has met the exile its protecting and has witnessed and validated the part.

A Few Other Notes on Exiles

Sometimes an exiled part wants its protector with it while you get to know it. That's *absolutely* fine. You want the exile to feel safe, and it may need the protector there in order to do so. Invite the protector to be with the exile in whatever way they would like to.

Sometimes protectors won't step back to allow us to meet exiles. They may be afraid that the exiled part will take over the system with its emotions, and they believe that that will be disastrous. Essentially, they're afraid that the exile will blend with you. If that happens, ask the exile not to overwhelm the system. Believe it or not, that works. Let the exile know that if they come on too strong, the protector is going to shut down the whole process, and they'll be by themselves again. Exiles don't want that, so they very often agree not to overwhelm you. Once that happens, the protectors are able to step back.

You can also ask the exile to take a step or two away from you so that you can remain unblended from it. This way, the part can still feel all its emotions but it's not making *you* feel those emotions. You can't be helpful if you're blended with it.

Protectors may also refuse to step back because they're afraid that you will reinjure the part, especially if they don't know you. If you're just starting IFS, it will take time for your parts to trust you. They need to see you coming back and checking in with them and the parts they're protecting. They may also be afraid that you're just trying to get rid of the part (which is *not* the case). When this happens, let the protector know that you value *all* your parts, and that your goal is to heal the part, not get rid of it. Also let the part know that you're here to connect with and help this exile let go of the pain it's carrying. You can also let the protector know that it can stay present and watch the process and jump in if it needs to. That usually lets them ease up a bit.

And finally, as we've discussed, exiles are carrying heavy emotions, and these emotions make sense given these parts' experiences. We aren't trying to help parts let go of every last emotion they're carrying—that's unrealistic. If a part is carrying sadness and grief related to loss, we wouldn't expect to let all of that go. But we can listen and validate the part and bring it to a safe space. Again, you may want to work with an IFS therapist to complete the unburdening process.

Your Turn: Connecting with an Exiled Part

Now that you understand more about this process, you can begin connecting with your exiles. You can follow the prompts below or visit http://www.newharbinger.com/57286 to download a recorded meditation that will guide you through the process. You may also print copies of this exercise to complete it more than once.

As with getting to know your protectors, make sure you have plenty of time to complete this process. Find a comfortable space and position, and try to limit distractions.

Step 1: Choose a target part.

My target part is: _____

Step 2: Find the part. Turn your attention inward. Notice whether this part is in or around your body. Once you've found the part, ask yourself these questions:

How do I see the part? Hear it? Feel it?

_____

_____

If I see it, what does it look like? What color or shape is it? How large or small is it?

_____

_____

_____

If I hear it, what is it saying?

_____

_____

_____

_____

If I feel it, what sensation am I experiencing?

_____

_____

_____

_____

If the part is outside my body, how close is it to me? (If it seems too close, ask it to settle back a little to give you space. If it's so far away that it's hard to connect to, you can either move toward it or ask it to come closer to you.)

_____

_____

Step 3: Embody Self-energy. Now that you've found the part, notice how you're feeling toward it. If you're feeling anything other than Self-energy, gently ask your other parts to give you some space. If any of them are unable to do that, they become the target part. Complete the process with that part.

Step 4: Befriend the part. Turn your curious Self-energy toward the part and ask it these questions:

Do you know who I am? (If not, let it know.)

_____

How old are you?

_____

How old do you think I am? (If the part doesn't know or thinks you're a different age, update it.)

_____

What would you like me to know about you? (Invite the part to share any stories, memories, feelings, or beliefs with you. Take your time and offer the part your compassionate Self-energy.)

_____

_____

_____

_____

What beliefs are you carrying about yourself based on your experiences?

_____

_____

_____

_____

Do you feel that I truly understand your experiences? Is there more that you'd like to tell me?

_____

_____

_____

_____

Step 5: Ask how you can help and check in.

What do you need from me?

_____

How can I be a resource to you?

_____

How often would you like me to check in with you? Again, the IFS community recommends checking in with exiles daily for three weeks, but if the part wants something different, that's okay.

_____

_____

Step 6: Reconnect with the protector part.

Let's go back to the protector part and ask it these questions:

What did you notice about my experience with the exile?

_____

_____

_____

How are you feeling toward the exile now?

_____

_____

How do you feel about your job at this point? What would it be like for you to step back a bit?

_____

_____

_____

Checking In

Take a few moments to reflect on what that process was like for you.

How was it for you to get to know an exile?

_____

_____

_____

_____

What did you learn from the part?

_____

_____

_____

What was surprising about what you learned?

_____

_____

_____

How are your other parts responding to this process? Are they excited? Confused? Relieved? Check inside to notice.

_____

_____

_____

Getting to know your exiles can be an emotional process, but I hope you now realize how these parts lead to your protectors either eating or restricting food and how much help and support that they need. Remember, your relationship with food is complicated. Eating and restricting is driven by a deeper process that involves your exiles, and if they aren't attended to, your eating patterns will be very difficult to change.

It may take time to sit with your exiles, listen to, and witness their stories. That's okay. Just connecting with your exiles and offering them compassion is huge and immensely valuable.

CHAPTER 6

What to Do When Firefighters Take Over

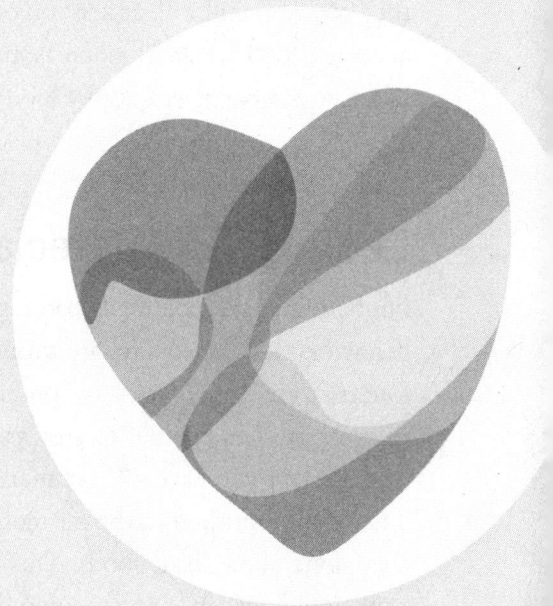

So far, you've gotten to know your Self and many of your parts. In this chapter, we're going to focus on your firefighters: what triggers them and what to do when they're active. I would love to say that once you get to know your firefighters, they'll never jump in and take over your system again...but they probably still will, at least on occasion. And that's not a bad thing! Remember, the goal is not to *never* use food for emotional reasons again. Sometimes it's just what your parts need. But once we get to know our parts, we can use food in a calmer, more aware manner.

Learning to Appreciate Your Firefighters

Firefighter parts get a really bad rap in our system and our culture. They're the parts who engage in behaviors that society says are wrong. Our manager parts have learned these messages well and therefore try to silence, control, or contain these parts. What happens then? Your firefighters have to jump in even stronger in order to push past your managers.

Let's say you have a lot of manager parts who engage in controlling or restricting what you eat. They make sure you never eat more calories than they think you should, they weigh you daily, and they don't allow "bad" foods. This is *not* an eating pattern that all your parts are on board with, so your firefighters are going to jump in any time they get the chance to get you to eat all the foods your managers don't let you eat.

Say you're at a birthday party and someone hands you a piece of cake. Those firefighters are going to say, "Yes! Finally!"—and possibly lead you back to the dessert table for more food, or take you to the nearest bakery on your way home to get even more cake. Since they finally have a chance to shove the managers aside, they may go for it big time.

This is why firefighters blend with you so quickly and strongly–they *need* to. They know that those managers are going to jump back in at some point, so they had better enjoy their freedom while it lasts. Firefighters also blend so quickly because they're soothing parts. They're truly trying to make other parts feel better. When the exiles they protect become triggered, firefighters jump in immediately to take care of them, and we need to show them our gratitude. Showing our firefighters appreciation goes a very long way to connecting with them, which allows them to soften.

Take a moment to jot down your thoughts about your firefighters.

_____

_____

_____

If you're noticing parts who are frustrated or annoyed by them, just take notice of them and ask them to settle back. And then thank those firefighters for all the hard work they do!

Let's Talk About Awareness

Awareness is a huge piece of our ultimate goal: Self-led eating. The more aware we are of who's leading us to food and why, the less likely we are to become blended with our firefighters. Being aware of our firefighters allows us to find out why they're feeling the need to swoop in.

Having awareness of your triggers and the parts involved gives you options in terms of how to respond to them. These options include:

Communication. Talk with your firefighters and the exiles they're protecting about how to potentially navigate people, places, and things differently so that your firefighters don't need to swoop in.

Planning. It's incredibly helpful to plan for triggering events when we can. A plan may include avoiding or leaving a triggering situation early so that your parts don't have to participate, or checking in with an exile before, during, and after the triggering event to let it know that you're there and see how you can be helpful.

Letting your parts off the hook. Believe it or not, we can let our parts know that they don't have to go to stressful events or be around people who trigger them. Yes, that actually works! You can let your parts know that *you* can handle the person or situation, and they don't even need to be there. Check in with your exiles before the event, and create a cozy, safe space for them to hang out in while you handle the event itself. Check in with them afterward as well.

Setting boundaries. Take the time to create Self-led boundaries around people, places, and things that trigger your firefighters. Do you really need to go to social events that make your parts uncomfortable? Do you really need to be around triggering people? Or are these, perhaps, your people-pleasing parts running the show?

Most of us have certain people, places, situations, or even conversation topics that feel threatening to our exiles and trigger our firefighters to jump in. For those with a history of trauma, even sounds or smells can be triggering. When our exiles get triggered, our firefighters jump in to soothe them by either eating or restricting (or engaging in other behaviors, but here we're just focusing on what they do with food).

To help us be more aware, we're going to spend some time identifying what has caused our firefighters to take over in the past. Take a moment to reflect on and answer these questions:

Remember a time when a firefighter took over. What had triggered the exile, and what was the exile feeling?

_____

_____

_____

Now, let's try to identify patterns. Who are the people in your life that tend to trigger your parts?

_____

_____

_____

What is it about these people that is triggering?

_____

_____

_____

In what circumstances or situations do you tend to feel triggered? (For example, is it difficult for you to go to your parents' house? Are there places that just make you uncomfortable? Are there certain situations, like large groups, that are difficult for you? Jot down any and all details.)

_____

_____

_____

_____

_____

_____

What else do you notice that triggers your parts?

_____

_____

_____

_____

_____

_____

_____

_____

Now that you've noticed some of your triggers, you can dive a little deeper and get to know the parts of you that react to them. Take a moment to review your responses to the questions above, and pick out the parts involved. For example, perhaps you've noticed that a sibling is triggering your parts. Get curious about why that is. Perhaps your sibling triggers parts of you that don't feel good enough or who felt ignored by your parents. Add these to your parts list and get to know them in the same way you've been getting to know your parts thus far.

What Foods Do My Firefighters Choose?

In addition to being aware of what people, places, and situations trigger your firefighters, it can be really helpful to know what foods they tend to steer you toward. Knowing that your firefighters lead you to sweets when they get triggered, for example, can really help you recognize their presence. I know that a firefighter is running the show when I'm heading for ice cream, so I do my best to check in with that part when I find myself at the freezer. Similarly, I know if I'm buying a box of mac 'n cheese, I've got a kid part who's looking for some comfort food. If you know the foods that your parts turn you to, you'll be tuned into your firefighters every time you find yourself grabbing these foods.

Take some time to make a list of the foods your firefighters tend to turn to:

_____

_____

_____

_____

_____

Just making that list has already increased your awareness and will help you pause and check in when you're reaching for these foods. Here's another way to use this awareness: put something in or around your trigger foods to cue you to check in with yourself when you're going to those foods. I did this years ago. My daughter loves M&Ms, and I kept a container in the house for her. Back when I was just getting to know my parts who turned me to food, I put a note inside the container to cue me to check in and see who was driving me to this food. When I saw the note, I stopped what I was doing and connected with the firefighter who wanted the M&Ms to find out what it needed. Sometimes I still ate the candy, but many times I didn't because I was able to give the part what it truly needed.

Similarly, there may be other behaviors you engage in when parts are triggered, such as exercising or using substances. It's helpful to check in with parts when you notice yourself engaging in these behaviors as well.

Now, make a list of other behaviors your firefighters tend to engage in:

_____

_____

_____

_____

_____

What Emotions Trigger My Firefighters?

As we've discussed, our exiles trigger our firefighters due to the intense emotions they carry. For example, a firefighter might jump in very strongly when an exiled part feels shame. Knowing that shame will likely lead to a firefighter jumping in is really helpful: you can now be on the lookout for shame, and Self can check in with that part before a firefighter jumps in.

Knowing what you're feeling can be difficult, as many people have never been taught to label their emotions. A feelings wheel, which organizes and categorizes a multitude of emotions, can help you pinpoint and label exactly what you're feeling. You can find a free one at https://feelingswheel.com.

Be on the lookout for the feelings that you know trigger your firefighters, and check in with the parts who are carrying them when they arise.

Now, let's gather everything you've learned about what triggers your firefighters and how they respond and add it to your Firefighter Awareness worksheet located on the following page. If you need more space, or additional copies, you can also find the worksheet at http://www.newharbinger.com/57286, you'll find a blank copy of this worksheet that you can download and print. Put your list where it can be easily seen to cue you to pause when you notice your triggers and/or your firefighters jumping in. For example, if one of the foods that your firefighters tend to love is in your pantry, put the list on the pantry door or somewhere else where you can see it easily. That way, when you're reaching for that food, you'll be cued to stop and check in.

Firefighter Awareness Worksheet

Notice the people, places, situations, and emotions that trigger your firefighters. Then, add the foods that they tend to turn you toward.

People: _____

_____

_____

_____

Places: _____

_____

_____

_____

Situations: _____

_____

_____

_____

Emotions: _____

_____

_____

_____

These are my firefighters' favorite foods: _____

_____

_____

Unblending from Your Firefighters

Now, let's talk about what to do when a firefighter takes over. Let's say one of your parts has been triggered, and a firefighter is heading for the ice cream. Because it's on your list of foods that firefighters turn to, you have a Post-it note on the ice cream that says "Check in." This guide will help you know what to do.

- Leave the room. It's much easier to connect to your parts when you aren't staring at their favorite food. Find somewhere quiet where you can check in.

- Ask the part to give you space so that you can notice it and connect with it.

- If you notice parts who are upset or frustrated at this part, ask them to step back and give you space.

- Find your Self-energy. Let the part know that you're open and curious toward it, and that you'd love to offer your help.

- Ask the part what's going on for it right now, and what led to it wanting food.

- Listen and validate the part. Let it know that you understand it was trying to be helpful.

- If you have time, get to know the part by moving through all of the steps from your Getting to Know a Protector Part worksheet or listen to the corresponding meditation.

- Ask the part how you can be helpful to it. Ask what it would need to feel calmer. Do your best to give it what it needs.

- Thank the part for all it does for you.

- Make the commitment to check in with the part later in the day or the next day to see how it's doing.

It takes time to get the hang of this process, and it's okay if it doesn't go smoothly at first. Offer your parts compassion and try it again. I promise you that the more you get to know your firefighters when they aren't active, and the more aware you become of your triggers, the easier this will all get. The above guide can also be found at http://www.newharbinger.com/57286—feel free to print it out and keep it easily available, or bring it up on your phone. At the same link, you'll also find a meditation you can use in these moments.

I hope this chapter has helped you become far more aware of your firefighters, what triggers them, and how to approach them when they start to take over. Keep in mind that noticing firefighters in the moment takes time and practice. Continue getting to know them, and I promise you, they will start to soften.

CHAPTER 7

The Principles of Intuitive Eating

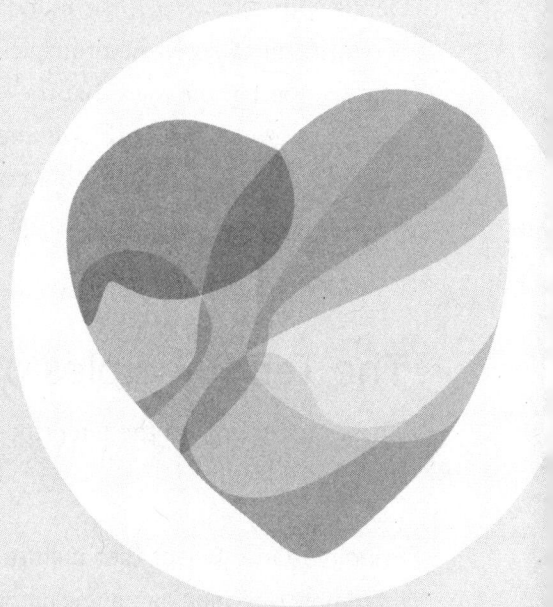

Up to now, we've been focusing on IFS and getting to know your parts. In this chapter, we're going to blend all that work with Intuitive Eating (IE), a practice that will help you tune into your body and respect and nourish it in the ways it needs. We'll focus on the principles of IE and how the model blends with IFS. To me, the foundation of IFS is essential to becoming an intuitive eater. It can be very difficult to apply the principles of IE without truly doing the work to understand *why* your parts relate to food in the ways that they do. Thankfully, you're already ahead of the game!

The primary goal of IE is *attunement*, which is the ability to tune into your body and give it what it needs. The ten principles that comprise IE all work toward that goal by guiding you either toward tuning into your body or removing what's blocking you from tuning into your body.

The Ten Principles of IE

These descriptions of the ten principles are each written through the lens of IFS to demonstrate how IFS and IE blend.

Principle One: Reject diet culture. Intuitive Eating is an anti-diet approach that recognizes how incredibly toxic and damaging diet culture is to all of us. Our parts have learned these toxic messages, and some have developed their roles based on them, but our Self does not support diet culture and recognizes the damage it does.

Principle Two: Honor your hunger. Keeping your body well fed not only leads to good health but also prevents polarization between restricting and eating parts. Parts that go to food are less likely to become triggered if your body is well nourished. Learning to notice your hunger cues is also a great way to begin building trust in your body and between Self and your parts.

Principle Three: Make peace with food. The founders of IE strongly suggest giving yourself unconditional permission to eat. This means there are no off-limits foods. Why? Because deprivation very often leads to eating. Allowing our parts to have any food they like leads to a decrease in polarization between restricting and binge eating.

Principle Four: Discover the satisfaction factor. The founders of IE believe that satisfaction is the hub of IE. It's incredibly important to consume food that is satisfying to all your parts as well as to your body. Using Self-led curiosity to notice such foods allows you to eat in ways that are beneficial to your whole system.

Principle Five: Feel your fullness. Checking in with your body's fullness cues is key, and so is noticing the parts of you who may talk you into ignoring those cues.

Principle Six: Challenge the food police. This principle looks a lot like IFS. The founders of IE introduce the "parts" that have taken in messages from diet culture and engage in rigid food rules. Luckily, you've already done this work!

Principle Seven: Cope with your emotions with kindness. This principle looks at ways you can approach emotional concerns without food. Again, you've already been doing that by connecting to your compassionate Self-energy and getting to know your parts.

Principle Eight: Respect your body. Remember that IE is not focused on weight loss, and neither is your Self. The negative beliefs and feelings you have toward your body are carried by parts, and we can help them let that go. IE wholeheartedly believes in treating your body with the respect it deserves, and so does IFS.

Principle Nine: Movement—Feel the difference. Some of our parts follow rigid rules about exercise, which can be damaging both physically and emotionally. This principle encourages you and your parts to engage in whatever movement you like without any rules and expectations.

Principle Ten: Honor your health—Gentle nutrition. I truly believe that our Self wants us to be healthy, and this principle provides basic nutritional advice on how to nurture our bodies well.

Thanks to IFS you're doing so much of this work already, so for now, we'll focus on these five principles: rejecting diet culture; honoring your hunger; feeling your fullness; making peace with food, and respecting your body (this principle will be covered in chapter 8).

Rejecting Diet Culture

Essentially, diet culture is the social value system that has created a hierarchy of acceptable bodies, with thin, white, straight, able ones at the top. This system uses a very narrow view of health and beauty, and considers some bodies to be more valuable, attractive, and deserving of respect. Diet culture also equates thinness to morality and health and promotes the idea that losing weight leads to increased social status.

Thanks to diet culture, we have the diet industry, which consists of diet and pharmaceutical companies, as well as weight loss–focused dietitians, wellness professionals, influencers, and personal trainers, all of whom buy into and contribute to the belief that weight loss is of utmost importance. The diet industry is a multibillion dollar industry that, according to businesswire.com (2023), made $75 billion in 2022.

And here's the deal: diets don't work. Research has consistently shown that about 95 percent of dieters regain all of their lost weight, typically within five years (Harrison 2021). Put another way, only about 5 percent of dieters lose a significant amount of weight and keep it off long-term. Would you get on a plane that had a 95 percent chance of crashing? Or see a surgeon who can promise you only a 5 percent chance of waking up? Of course not! But the diet industry has been such an evil genius that when your diet doesn't work and you regain your weight (and possibly more), you blame *yourself*. Not the diet. Which of course leads your parts to feel shame. Hopeless. Not good enough.

And those feelings very often take you right back to dieting. And since you now understand parts more, you know why, right? Your protector parts work toward weight loss as a way of protecting your exiles who don't feel good enough. And that will keep happening until you work with your parts to understand them, unburden them, and help them shift their roles.

Let's consider how your parts think about and respond to diet culture:

What is your current awareness of the dangers and pitfalls of diet culture? If you were aware of the above information, where did you learn it? If not, what questions do you hope to answer?

_____

_____

_____

_____

What does the discussion of dieting bring up for you? What feelings do your parts have about this topic?

_____

_____

_____

_____

The Physical Damage of Dieting

Our bodies don't like dieting because dieting is a form of starvation, plain and simple. Our bodies, obviously, don't want to starve—they're wired to stay alive. That's a good thing! Because of this innate drive, dieting wreaks havoc on our systems. The founders of IE describe the physical damage caused by restrictive diets (Tribole and Resch 2020). They cite research suggesting that dieting:

- causes the body to retain more fat when you resume a more regular eating pattern;

- decreases your metabolism;

- increases binge eating and cravings;

- increases the risk of premature death and heart disease (This is largely related to weight cycling, the chronic pattern of weight loss and regain, which puts you at twice the risk of dying of heart disease.); and causes satiety cues to atrophy, possibly leading you to eat larger meals.

Think back to your experience of dieting. Which, if any, of these symptoms have you experienced? Describe any other physical symptoms you've experienced.

_____

_____

_____

_____

_____

_____

_____

_____

The Psychological and Emotional Damage of Dieting

Not surprisingly, the damage of dieting is not only physical—it's psychological and emotional as well. Research has shown that dieters are more likely to develop an eating disorder than nondieters. One such study showed that women who dieted moderately were five times more likely to develop an eating disorder and those who practiced extreme restriction were eighteen times more likely to develop an eating disorder than those who did not diet (Patton et al. 1999). As someone who treats people with eating disorders, I can tell you that I've never had a client who hasn't dieted. Never.

Additionally, during a landmark 1992 National Institutes of Health Weight Loss and Control Conference, experts reported that dieting is correlated with feelings of failure, lower self-esteem, and social anxiety. Experts further noted that dieting may cause stress or cause the dieter to become vulnerable to its effects (Tribole and Resch 2020).

I've never met a dieter who felt comfortable in their own skin. All my clients have dieted, and they've all struggled with parts who don't feel good enough, hate their bodies, and feel shame about their eating behaviors. They tend to experience anxiety and depression related to food and their body, and they constantly compare themselves to others. Dieting has never once solved these issues for them, at least not in the long run. I'm guessing it didn't for you either.

Take a moment to reflect on how you've felt while dieting in the past. How was the experience for your parts? What did they like about dieting? What did they not like? Did it give them what they were hoping for?

_____

_____

_____

_____

_____

_____

_____

_____

How Do You Stop Dieting?

Just because you may know why, logically, you should reject diet culture doesn't mean that it's easy to just stop dieting. Remember, our parts have internalized messages from diet culture that they've been hearing their whole lives, and they may still wholeheartedly believe them. They're very nervous about no longer dieting because dieting is their job, and it serves a purpose: protecting other parts. These parts won't know how to help you and your parts if they aren't dieting. Our goal is to get to know all these parts and give them updated information (that is, that your Self does not believe in diet culture, that dieting usually leads to weight gain, and so on) and to help them feel safe enough to shift their roles and let go of dieting.

Let's start updating your parts now. We'll start by finding parts who are carrying diet culture beliefs. Take a look at the diet culture facts above and notice all of your parts' responses to this information. These will be parts to get to know individually and educate about the truth concerning dieting, so note them below and add them to your parts list.

_____

_____

_____

_____

_____

For now, we'll update them as a group. Invite all those parts to join you in a comfortable space, perhaps around a nice table or sitting outside under a beautiful tree. Once these parts are there, let them know that you'd like to talk with them about the misinformation they've been told about bodies, their body, food, society, and so on. Let them know that you—your Self— knows that these were lies. Give them some examples of this information, and just notice how they're responding. Take a few minutes to do this, and note below how these parts responded to this new information.

_____

_____

_____

_____

My guess is that there were parts who had difficulty accepting this information. That's completely understandable. It's difficult for parts to realize they've been lied to, possibly by an important person in your life. Parts may also be concerned that if this information is true, they may need to change what they've been doing, which is scary. Or they may fear that your system will decide to stop dieting, which may lead to such consequences as weight gain, loss of (perceived) control regarding food, or isolation. (You may be the only person you know who isn't dieting—that's really difficult.) We want to approach all these parts with compassionate Self-energy.

Now list the parts of you who are having difficulty accepting this new information about dieting. Notice what they're saying about why this is difficult, and offer them your compassion. Then, add them to your parts list to get to know them later.

_____

_____

_____

_____

_____

_____

_____

Now let's focus on the parts of you that use dieting to protect other parts. These are likely managers, and you may already have gotten to know some of them. Head back to chapter 2 and look at the Dieter/Restrictor parts you noted. If you haven't already done so, add these parts to your parts list and get to know them like you would any other manager part. Again, dieting for these parts is a way to protect exiles, and they won't feel safe enough to stop dieting until you've gotten to know them and unburdened the exile they're protecting.

And finally, take a moment to think about what it would be like to stop dieting. Pay particular attention to any fear or anxiety that comes up when you think about it. Some of these parts may be managers who engage in dieting, and some may be parts who just like dieting itself or like its results. And some may be fearful of the potential consequences of no longer dieting (for example, weight gain or loss of control over food). It's imperative that you get to know these parts and address their concerns, or they will continue to keep you engaged in the dieting process.

List any thought, feeling, or bodily sensation that comes up when you think about no longer dieting. Then, list these as parts on your parts list and get to know them at a later time.

_____

_____

_____

_____

_____

_____

_____

Tuning Into Hunger and Fullness Cues

Do you typically notice when you're hungry? Or do you eat by the clock? Do you notice when you're full? And if so, do you stop or continue eating? Jot down your responses to these questions.

_____

_____

_____

_____

_____

_____

Many people have difficulty tuning into their hunger and fullness cues. There are a few reasons for that, and many of them involve parts. Let's start with the fact that many of us aren't taught to notice these cues. If you grew up in a household where breakfast was at 8:00 a.m., lunch was at noon, and dinner was at 6:00 p.m., hunger cues probably had nothing to do with when you ate. Similarly, how often did someone encourage you to check in with your body and notice how hungry or full you were? Probably never. Or at least rarely. If you weren't taught or encouraged to tune into these cues, why would you notice them now?

A second reason you may not notice these cues is that most of us tend to lead busy lives. Taking the time to slow down, relax, and check in with your body while eating is a luxury that many of us don't have. Or at least we don't take the time to have it. You might be someone who has so much to attend to throughout the day that it's incredibly difficult to slow down and notice your body's cues. You may also have parts who *keep* you really busy as a way of protecting you. Look back at chapter 2 to see if you checked off the box under "The Doer." If you did, write those parts below. If you didn't, check in with your system now and see if you can find any. List them here, and try to notice why they might be so busy. Then add them to your parts list.

_____

_____

_____

Another reason that you may not notice your hunger and fullness cues is that you have parts who are blocking that process. There are a few reasons why parts may block your ability to notice hunger and fullness cues, the first being food scarcity. Certainly, if you're currently experiencing or have ever experienced food scarcity, your parts may have blocked your hunger cues because they were just too painful, which absolutely makes sense. How can you get through your day if you're constantly feeling hungry? If you've ever experienced food scarcity and have difficulty noticing your hunger cues, add blocking parts to your list of parts.

Maybe you have parts who tend to restrict the types of food you eat, and when you're finally eating one of those forbidden foods, your parts say, "Forget it! I'm eating it all!" In that case, there might be parts who are disconnecting you from your body because they're finally getting the food they enjoy and they don't want that to stop, so they block you from feeling full.

Parts may also block the connection to your body (and therefore your hunger and fullness cues) because connecting to your body is painful. If you're someone who's experienced trauma related to your body, it makes sense that your parts are keeping you disconnected from it in order to help you feel safe and not relive your trauma.

It may also be painful for some parts to connect to your body if your body isn't functioning at the level your parts would like. Perhaps you have a medical or physical issue that causes pain or hinders your life in some way. Your parts may not want you to really experience that issue and therefore they disconnect you from your body.

And finally, parts may disconnect you from your body if they don't like your body. As you read earlier, many, if not most, of us have parts who are critical toward our body. If these parts are feeling really negatively toward your body, they may just disconnect you from it. It's their way of pretending your body isn't there.

Noticing Your Hunger Cues

A great way to start noticing your hunger cues is first to describe how hunger feels in your body. Answer these questions about your hunger, and come back to them periodically and add to your responses as you get to know your hunger cues more fully.

How do you know you're hungry?

_____

_____

_____

_____

In what parts of your body does hunger tend to appear? (This might be your stomach, head, mouth, or any other area.)

_____

_____

_____

_____

How does hunger feel in those parts of your body?

_____

_____

_____

_____

How do your parts tend to respond to hunger? (For example, are they excited to eat? Are they scared of feeling hungry?)

_____

_____

_____

_____

_____

If you're having any difficulty answering these questions, you may have parts who have been blocking your hunger cues. When you have some time, invite those parts to be present with you. Check in with your system and ask who might have fears and concerns about feeling hunger. And then just listen. If you have blocking parts, they'll likely make themselves known. Take the time to get to know these parts and come back to this section at a later time.

If you were able to answer only some of these questions, just remain curious. Focus closely on your body the next time you notice any twinge of hunger, and try to expand your awareness. Again, return to the above questions and flesh out your responses.

The Hunger Rating Scale

If you feel like you have a good grasp of when you're hungry, the next step is to notice your hunger levels. The scale that follows can help you do just that. You may have seen or used hunger rating scales in the past. Many of them go from 1 to 10, which honestly confuses my parts—that's just too many numbers to choose from! What is the subtle difference between a 4 and a 5? Here the scale is simplified to rate your hunger from 1 to 7.

As you can see, ideally you would begin eating at a 2 and stop at a 6. But since we no longer have hard-and-fast rules about that (right?), this is more of a guideline. Obviously, there'll be times when that doesn't happen, and that's okay. But since we're working toward tending to our bodies and respecting what they need, we want to respect hunger and fullness cues. For the most part (as the founders of IE remind us), you're going to eat when you're hungry and stop when you're full. But obviously, there are times when that just won't happen, and you're not going to beat yourself up about that anymore.

If this hunger rating scale feels too diet-y to you, don't use it. I don't want any of your parts to feel as though you're heading back into another diet framework. You can still work on noticing hunger and fullness cues without using a rating scale. Just focus on learning your cues and checking in with your body frequently throughout the day to notice your hunger level.

For now, just notice where your hunger falls on the rating scale as often as you can when you're wanting food. Print a copy from http://www.newharbinger.com/57286 and keep it nearby so that you can use it frequently. We'll talk more about how to use it in chapter 9.

Hunger Rating Scale

1—I feel painfully hungry, my stomach hurts.

2—I feel hungry, my stomach is growling, I feel ready to eat. (Ideally, begin eating now.)

3—I'm slightly hungry; I could eat but it's not necessary.

4—I'm neutral, not feeling hungry or full.

5—I feel slightly full but could eat a few more bites.

6—I feel full, satisfied, comfortable. (Ideally, stop eating now.)

7—I feel stuffed, my clothes are tight, I definitely ate too much.

Noticing Your Fullness Cues

Tuning into fullness cues may be difficult for all the reasons we've discussed, and also because it's very likely that you have parts who talk you into continuing to eat even if you're already full.

Let's start getting to know your fullness cues by describing them and how they feel in your body. Take the time to answer these questions about fullness. And again, come back to them periodically and add to your responses as you get to know your fullness cues more fully.

How do you know you're full?

_____

_____

_____

_____

_____

In what parts of your body does fullness tend to appear? (This might be your stomach, head, mouth, or any other area.)

_____

_____

_____

_____

_____

How does fullness feel in these parts of your body?

_____

_____

_____

_____

_____

How do your parts tend to respond to fullness? (Do they respect those cues and stop eating? Do they tell you to keep going?)

_____

_____

_____

_____

_____

If you answered the last question with "Yes, my parts tend to keep me eating after I'm full," you're not alone. In my experience, eating to the point of discomfort is more often about parts who keep you going rather than not being attuned to your fullness cues. And a great way to start noticing parts is to start noticing the thoughts you have while eating. Do any of these statements sound familiar?

- This food is delicious. I don't want to stop.

- I almost never get to eat this, so I'm going to eat it until it's gone.

- It's only a few more bites—I'll just keep going.

- I need to clean my plate.

- There's not enough here to save it—I'll eat it because I can't waste food.

These are examples of different parts who keep you eating for various reasons. And we want to get to know them too! If you're someone who tends to eat past the point of fullness, take a few moments to think about what parts are saying to you while you're eating. Write them down and add these parts to your parts list. Continue to notice these types of parts while you're eating to be sure you have a complete list.

_____

_____

_____

_____

_____

_____

Making Peace with Food

This is one of my favorite principles in IE. And the founders summarize it well by saying:

> "Call a truce, stop the food fight! Give yourself unconditional permission to eat. If you tell yourself that you can't or shouldn't have a particular food, it can lead to intense feelings of deprivation that build into uncontrollable cravings and, often, bingeing. When you finally 'give in' to your forbidden foods, eating will be experienced with such intensity, it will usually result in Last Supper overeating and overwhelming guilt" (Tribole and Resch 2020).

Does that sound familiar? Have you ever had the experience of cutting out a certain food and then feeling so deprived that you eat it with reckless abandon? This cycle is extremely common, and there are many reasons for it. One involves polarized parts. Remember that we often have two parts or two groups of parts on opposite sides (such as a bingeing part and a restricting part) and that when one side gets activated, the other side also gets activated and has to outdo the first side. So, when you restrict, it actually triggers your binge eating parts.

Intuitive Eating encourages you to escape this restrict-binge cycle by giving yourself unconditional permission to eat. No foods are off-limits.

Check in with your system and notice how your parts are responding to the idea of giving yourself unconditional permission to eat. My guess is they range from very excited to terrified! Please let all your parts know that you aren't just jumping into this with reckless abandon. There's a process that we'll be following.

_____

_____

_____

_____

_____

The Importance of Habituation

Have you ever purchased a new car? Or at least one that's new to you? For the first few weeks (or even months), you probably found it exciting to get into that car and drive. It's almost like when you first got your driver's license. But after a while, it just becomes that thing with tires that takes you from point A to point B. Driving that car isn't exciting any more. This is because you've habituated to driving it.

Habituation is the process of adapting to an experience after repeated exposure to it, leading to a decrease in pleasure of that experience. We habituate to all kinds of things—even people. Think about when you first met a new friend or your partner. It was really exciting, wasn't it! They were so interesting, and it was really fun getting to know them. But after some time passes, although they're still wonderful, being with them often doesn't have the same level of excitement it once did.

The same thing happens with food. Let's try an experiment: Think of your favorite food. It may be one you eat frequently, or one you never allow yourself to eat. Try to notice the aroma, the taste, and the texture of that food. You might be noticing yourself feeling excited about it just by thinking about it. Now, imagine eating that food every single day for the next year. How do you think you would feel by day 365? Or even day 102? I doubt it would be the same level of excitement as you had on day one.

This is the process of habituation. Even your favorite food loses its luster if you eat it every single time you want it. *Systematic habituation* is the process of eating a forbidden food whenever you want it with the goal of habituating to it (Tribole and Resch 2025). We'll be using the foundation of this process and adding some IFS to it. Once you've habituated to a food, it doesn't call your name with the same level of intensity or frequency as it had previously. And you eventually prove to yourself that that food does not need to be forbidden—that you can keep it right on your counter and eat it only when a part really wants it.

Systematic Habituation

Let's dive into the process of systematic habituation and get to know the parts involved. You'll choose one food to habituate to. It's important that you *eat the exact same food each time*. Let's say you'd like to habituate to ice cream. Be sure that you eat the same brand and flavor every single time, as varying flavors will interfere with habituation. Once you feel like the food no longer has the same pull for you, move on to another food.

The process is described below. At http://www.newharbinger.com/57286, you'll find a worksheet that you can download to use with each new food.

1. Choose a time when you are not likely to be too hungry (so that your eating parts aren't tempted to eat the forbidden food too quickly and without attending to it).

2. Next, choose a specific food. Again, be sure that you eat the exact same food until you habituate to it.

3. Decide where you will eat the food. It may be helpful to start the process by eating the food outside your home. Choose whatever feels safest for your parts.

   ☐ Kitchen

   ☐ Dining room

   ☐ Another room in your home

   ☐ Outside your home

   ☐ Other: _____

Checking In During the Eating Process

Before. Notice all the parts who come up for you when you sit down to eat this food.

During. Notice the taste, texture, and aroma of the food. Is the food meeting your expectation? Check in with your parts and notice how they're experiencing the food.

After. How was the experience of eating this food? Was the taste as enjoyable as you had expected? Notice how your parts are feeling now that you've eaten it.

Continue to eat this food when you want to until you can walk by it and not feel the need to eat it. Once that happens, move on to another forbidden food.

Generally speaking, the more you do this, the easier it gets because your parts finally trust that you're allowing yourself to eat foods that were previously forbidden. It can take some time for your parts to trust that you'll no longer restrict these foods. Once they trust you, the habituation process goes much faster.

If this exercise feels too difficult to do at this point, that's okay. Don't start it if your parts are scared. Continue working with the parts who are fearful of it, and once they soften, give it a try. It may be helpful to start by choosing to eat the food outside your home. That would mean that whenever you want it, you allow yourself to go get it. If that feels safer, that's completely fine. Then advance the process by bringing the food into your home.

It's important to note that you don't need to keep all foods that you've habituated to in your house. Sure, it's great to know that food doesn't call to you very strongly any more, but you don't need to prove that to yourself daily by having these foods around. There are plenty of foods I don't keep in my house because it's just too easy for me to walk by and grab them, and not even notice I'm doing it. To me, it's not worth keeping them around. *However*, my parts also know that I will go get a food that I really want (after checking in with the part who really wants it). My parts know that I have *no* foods that are off-limits (although there are many foods that I don't eat often or at all because they don't agree with me), and they don't need me to keep them around.

If You're Feeling Overwhelmed...

We've covered a lot in this chapter alone, and certainly in this workbook so far. You may have parts who are feeling overwhelmed by all the parts you're discovering. That's completely normal. I often have clients who start out thinking that we're going to get to know two or three parts and be done with it. They're shocked to discover how complicated it all is (again, this is why it's been so difficult to change up until now). Check in with your overwhelmed parts and let them know they are not the ones who need to be doing all of this work. *You (Self)* are. And you are more than happy to do it. And remind your parts that this is a marathon and not a sprint. There is no expectation that you'll get to know each and every part in your eating system, and there's no deadline to finish this work by. Just take your time and stay curious. Slow and steady wins the race!

CHAPTER 8

Developing Body Respect

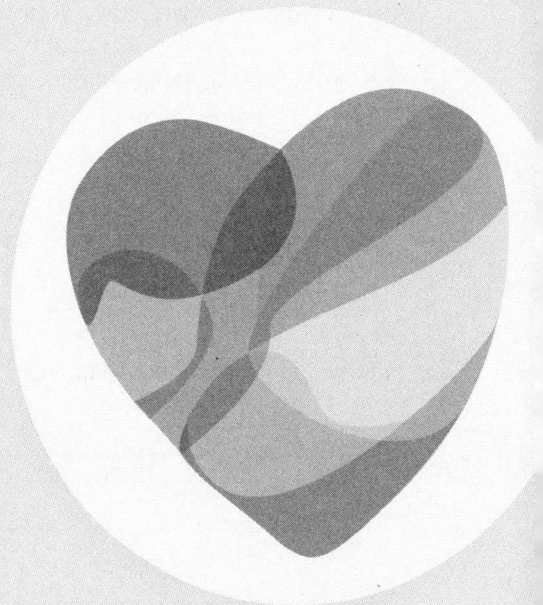

Before we get in to the work of developing body respect, let's go back to the beginning. At the end of the introduction to this workbook, I asked you how you would describe your current relationship with your body, and how you would like that to change. Please take a moment to answer those questions a second time and write down your responses here:

How would you describe your current relationship with your body?

_____

_____

_____

How would you like that to change?

_____

_____

_____

Now, glance back at your original answers to those two questions and ask yourself:

What, if anything, is different in your responses? What has changed for you?

_____

_____

_____

_____

There may not be much difference at this point, and that's okay—we'll work on that! But you may have also noticed at least a small change in how you regard your body. Your parts may have softened slightly when they think about your body, and much of that is likely due to the new information they've learned, the parts you've met, and connecting to your Self-energy.

Your Self and Your Body

What if I said to you that you—your Self—loves your body? Make a list of every part who just came up right now.

_____

_____

_____

_____

_____

_____

_____

_____

My guess is, you have parts who don't believe that for a second. They're saying, "That's not true. That's not possible. My Self knows that I need to change. I need to lose weight." Excuse my bluntness here, but those parts are incorrect.

Here's the thing about body shame and hating your body: it's 100 percent learned. Our culture tells us from day one that only a certain type of body is attractive, valuable, and worthwhile. And it even tells us that the bodies that match the ideal *still* aren't good enough. In other words, every body is flawed. Every body needs to be fixed in some way. We learn these messages from a very young age, and we see these messages daily. Some of us have gotten very specific messages from parents, partners, medical professionals, and others that our bodies are wrong. All of these messages translate into body shame and body hatred.

None of that body shame and hatred is authentic to you. You didn't create it. And your Self doesn't believe it.

This can be difficult to accept for many of your parts. The messages about bodies in our culture are so pervasive and insidious that we don't even recognize them as messages—our parts think they're facts. Large bodies can't run? Yep, that's a fact. All thin bodies are healthy? Yep, makes total sense. Able bodies are more valuable? Sure, totally agree. Except that *none* of that is true. And our Self knows it.

Because our parts believe the messages from diet culture, it's often difficult to unblend from them. Again, they think these messages are facts, and our parts think that Self agrees. I can't tell you how often clients tell me that they hate their body. When I suggest that we get curious about the part who said that, they say, "That's not a part—that's me." These parts have taken in messaging about bodies so deeply that they think our Self believes these messages. I assure you, it does not.

Let me give you an example of this. If you were a fly on the wall of my office on any given day, you would hear something like this:

Client: I really need to lose weight. I'm just not healthy, and I can't stand myself at this weight.

Me: How about we get curious about the part who just said that?

Client: That's not a part, that's me!

Me: I know that you think it's you—you've been lied to by diet culture your whole life about bodies. But I promise you, that's not you. That's a part.

Client: No, it's not. That's me.

Me: Can you humor me for just a minute? How about we get curious about this and see if it's you or if it's a part.

Client: Sure, but I'm telling you, it's me.

Me: When you hear the words "I really need to lose weight," where do you notice that?

Client: It's in my chest. It feels heavy.

Me: Great. Put your attention on that, and notice how you're feeling toward that heaviness.

Client: I agree with it. I think it's true.

Me: Okay. Can the part who thinks it's true step back?

Client: Yeah, it can.

Me: Great. Thank it for doing that. Put your attention back on that heaviness. How are you feeling toward it?

Client: I feel sad for it.

Me: Okay. Does that sad part need anything from you, or can it step back so you can get to know this part?

Client: It can step back.

Me: Great. Thank it for doing that. Put your attention back on that heaviness. How are you feeling toward it now?

Client: Open and curious.

Me: Great. Does the part know you're there?

Client: No.

Me: Okay. Let it know you're there, and let it know who you are.

Client: Okay. It knows I'm there now.

Me: Great. Ask it to tell you whatever it would like you to know about itself.

Client: It says that it's hard being in my body at this size. My body aches. And it's hard to find clothes that fit.

Me: Yeah, I get that. Let it know that you understand how hard that is.

Client: Okay. It's relieved to hear that I understand.

Me: I bet it is. What else would it like you to know?

Client: That it's also tired of trying so hard to lose weight. It never works. And that's so disappointing.

Me: Yes. I'm sure it is. Invite the part to tell you more about how disappointing that is.

Client: It's telling me how hard it is to get its hopes up, work really hard, and then nothing. It's also saying that it feels sad for my body because it's been trying to change it so much. It feels bad about that.

Me: Let it know that you really hear that. And I wonder if it would be helpful to tell your body that.

Client: Yeah, I think it would.

Can you see how this part, who was adamant that it was Self, is really a part? By getting curious, we can ask parts to unblend from Self and recognize them as parts who have learned a very insidious message about bodies.

What parts came up for you when you read this exchange? Does the exchange resonate with you?

_____

_____

_____

_____

How are your parts feeling about this concept that negative body image always comes from parts and isn't authentic to you?

_____

_____

_____

_____

_____

Exploring Messages About Bodies

Messages about bodies are delivered to us in a variety of ways. You may have received direct statements from others about your body, such as a parent telling you that you need to lose weight or peers bullying you about your size. But you may have also received more indirect messages through such things as watching how a parent spoke about or treated their own body, witnessing negative comments or actions from one person toward another regarding their body, or hearing negative comments made about strangers' bodies.

Please take time to answer these questions about messages you've received.

What messages have you received from parents, friends, and/or significant others about your body throughout the course of your life?

_____

_____

_____

_____

What message have you received from parents, friends, and/or significant others about bodies in general throughout the course of your life?

_____

_____

_____

_____

What messages have you received about your body from health professionals, such as physicians, dietitians, therapists, or trainers?

_____

_____

_____

_____

What messages have you received from diet culture and the wider society about bodies in general?

_____

_____

_____

_____

_____

How have all these messages impacted your relationship with your body?

_____

_____

_____

_____

_____

Mapping Your Parts

Parts who have thoughts and feelings about your body are typically managers and exiles, although there can be firefighters as well. The managers who are critical of your body or who want to change it are protecting exiles who don't feel good enough, who feel shame, or who feel unlovable. These managers have learned that one way to receive love and validation in our culture is to look a certain way and to have a certain body. Therefore, they believe if they just achieve that, your exiled parts will automatically feel good enough.

Unfortunately, though, that's just not accurate. Achieving a certain size may feel good for a while, but that doesn't heal our exiles. They'll continue to carry their negative feelings and beliefs until we unburden them.

Exiles who hold negative feelings about your body are often carrying feelings of shame about your body and the belief that your body isn't good enough the way it is. They've taken on the messaging given to them by diet culture. They may have also had firsthand experience of being bullied about your body, or have received explicit negative messages about your body. If you're someone who's experienced any type of trauma or abuse toward or about your body, these exiles are also carrying the feelings and memories of those experiences.

Distinguishing between managers and exiles can be difficult, especially when it comes to parts who have feelings toward your body (because these feelings are usually quite intense and blend quickly). As a rule of thumb, managers are typically the ones trying to change you, while exiles are the ones typically carrying the feelings about your body. Remember that you don't need to know if the part is a manager or an exile because we always begin the process of getting to know our parts in the same way. We find out what type of part it is when we ask about its job. Managers have jobs, exiles don't.

It's imperative that you're able to approach these parts with Self-energy, which can be difficult since parts have such strong feelings toward your body. One easy way to tell if you're blended with a part is to notice if you're feeling anything at all negative toward your body, or if you're feeling the need to change your body. If the answer is yes, you're in a part. *Any negative feeling or desire to change your body is coming from a part, not Self.*

Listing Your Parts

To get to know the parts of you that have feelings toward your body, we're going to go about it in the same way you've been getting to know the parts who use food for various reasons. And we'll start with noticing your thoughts. My guess is that you have numerous thoughts about your body—those are parts. Examples of these thoughts include:

- I need to lose weight.

- I hate my body—it's not good enough.

- I can't do anything until my body changes.

- Why can't my body be like hers?

- My body is disgusting.

Take a moment to notice all of the thoughts (parts) that come up for you when you think about your body. List them here and then transfer them to your parts list.

_____

_____

_____

_____

_____

Visualizing Your System

In addition to listing the parts who have feelings toward your body, it may be helpful to map them. We discussed how to do this in chapter 4. Feel free to use the blank map pages found at http://www. newharbinger.com/57286 or to draw each of your parts. Here's an example of what a map may look like:

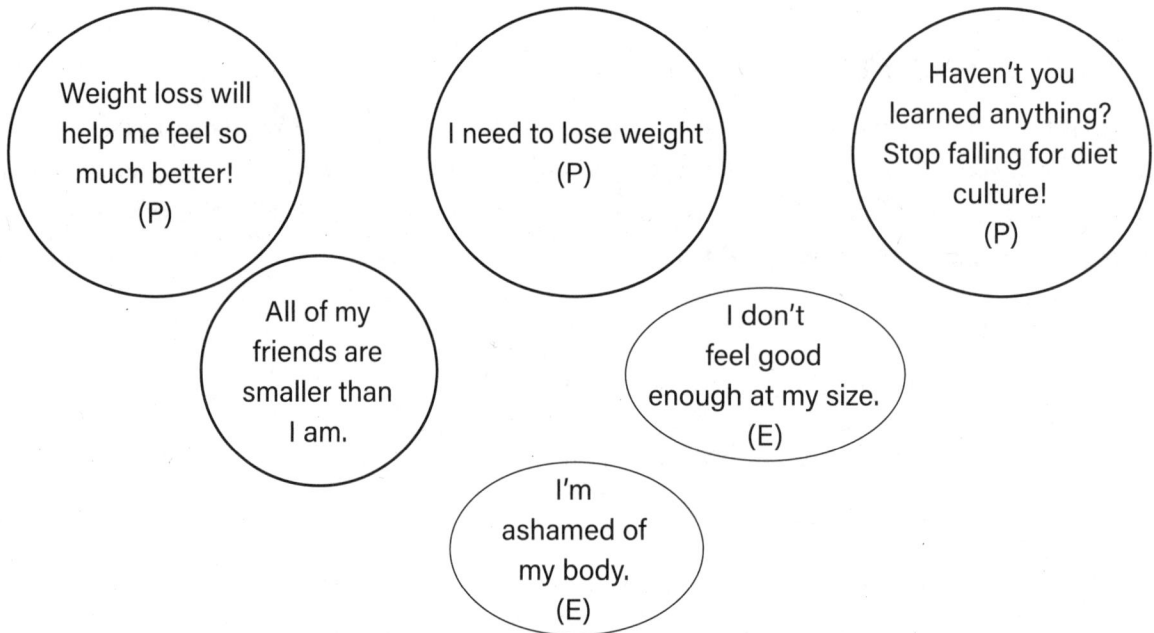

Weight loss will help me feel so much better! (P)

I need to lose weight (P)

Haven't you learned anything? Stop falling for diet culture! (P)

All of my friends are smaller than I am.

I don't feel good enough at my size. (E)

I'm ashamed of my body. (E)

Let's say this example is my system. As you can see, there are three pretty strong protector parts with thoughts and feelings about my body (the larger circles at the top). Two think it needs to change, and one is saying "Come on, haven't you learned anything from all you've read about diet culture yet? I don't want to keep dieting." (That one is polarized with the part in the middle). There are three other parts, two of whom seem to be exiles and one could be a protector or an exile.

Getting to Know a Part

From here, you're going to use the exact same process you've already been using to get to know your parts. This process should look very familiar to you by this point, so I'll just give you the highlights.

Step 1: Take a look at your list or your map and choose your target part. Select a part who doesn't seem overwhelming to you and that you have some Self-energy toward. As we did previously, it may be helpful to start with a protector instead of an exile.

My target part is: _____

Step 2: Once you're comfortable, turn your attention inward. Notice where the part is, in or around your body. Focus on bodily sensations or what the part might be saying to you. Remember that the part may be outside your body.

Step 3: Notice how you feel toward the part. If you're blended with another part, ask that part to step back. Once it does, place your attention on the target part and ask again. Continue this process until you know that your Self is present with the target part. Remember that this can be tricky with parts who have feelings toward your body. Other parts tend to think that those parts are Self—they are not. If you're having any difficulty getting to your Self-energy, that means that there are many parts with strong feelings about your body, and some (or all) may be having a hard time stepping back. Just try to notice all these parts, and come back to this at another time.

Step 4: Turn your curious Self-energy toward the part and ask it all the questions outlined in chapter 4. Use one of the worksheets or the guided meditation found at http://www.newharbinger.com/57286. I suggest using the Connecting with an Exiled Part exercise if you're not sure whether the part is a manager or an exile.

Step 5: If the part is a manager (that is, it has a job), ask it what it needs from you and who it's protecting. If it's able to tell you, ask it to introduce you to that part and start the process over with the exile as the target part. If the part is an exile, spend time getting to know it and validate its experiences. Ask it how you can be helpful.

Step 6: Ask the part how often it would like you to check in with it, and make a realistic plan to do so.

Once you've completed this, reflect on your experience.

What was that process like for you? Notice any and all thoughts, feelings, and parts who come up for you.

_____

_____

_____

_____

_____

_____

_____

_____

Developing Body Respect with IE

Body respect comes in two forms: making your body comfortable and responding to its basic needs (Tribole and Resch 2020). Focusing on these two aspects includes engaging in such activities as

eating when you're hungry;

dressing your body comfortably and in a style you enjoy;

moving comfortably and engaging in activity that your body likes;

setting boundaries in terms of physical touch;

no longer comparing your body to others;

doing your best to notice and stop body-bashing;

being realistic about your weight; and

focusing on what your body can do instead of what it looks like.

Some (or most) of that might seem daunting. You may have heard some parts say, "That's impossible!" But remember, those are parts. Your Self already has respect for your body. Take a moment to review the ideas above and jot down all of the parts who seem to be responding to it. These are parts to get to know at a later time, so add them to your parts list.

_____

_____

_____

_____

_____

What's Your Plan?

In addition to getting to know your parts (the most important piece of this work), it can be helpful to work toward some of the above activities. Maybe you'd like to focus on dressing your body comfortably. Make a plan for going shopping, and be sure to buy clothes that you really like and that fit well. Perhaps you'd like to focus on movement you enjoy. Make a plan for trying a new activity or returning to an old favorite.

Take some time to choose two or three of these activities (or come up with your own) and think about how you'll be implementing them. Check in with your parts to see what activities they'd like to focus on first, and create a realistic plan that most of your parts can support:

I'd like to focus on these two or three activities:

_____

_____

_____

_____

_____

Here's how I'm going to do it:

_____

_____

_____

_____

_____

_____

_____

_____

_____

Be sure to check in with your parts when engaging in these behaviors to see how they're feeling about it. If they need you to change something—or slow it down a bit—that's fine. Be open and curious about their feedback and experience, and work with them to figure out what's comfortable and beneficial for them.

To Weigh or Not?

One of the questions I often get from clients is whether they should weigh themselves. Honestly, I advise against it. Almost always, nothing good comes from weighing yourself. And the number itself actually means nothing. It's just a number, but our parts make a lot of meaning out of it. I tell my clients that if you're able to step on a scale, look at the number, and think, *Eh—whatever*, then fine—weigh yourself (although I'm not sure why you would). But if you can't, it's probably a good idea to try at the very least to weigh yourself less frequently.

How do you get to that point? Get to know the parts of you who want to step on the scale as well as the parts who are terrified of no longer weighing your body. If you just try to stop weighing yourself, that likely won't last. Remember, behavior change without understanding doesn't work. It's imperative that you explore this issue of weighing yourself and get to know the parts involved. Take a moment to answer these questions:

How often do you tend to weigh yourself?

_____

For how long have you been weighing yourself this frequently?

_____

If you remember why you began weighing yourself, please describe your reasons.

_____

_____

_____

_____

How do you typically feel when you step on the scale? (The response you get will be from parts—add them to your parts list.)

_____

_____

_____

When you think of no longer weighing yourself, what parts come up for you? Add these to your parts list.

_____

_____

_____

Let's Talk About Weight Loss (Again)

Most of us have, and will always have, parts who are concerned about weight and body size. But again, our Self doesn't care about the number on the scale. We must focus on healing our relationships with food and our bodies and let our body land where it's going to land. That sounds so simple, doesn't it?

Letting go of the goal of weight loss is difficult for most people, but it can be done. And of course, it's all about getting to know your parts. Check in with your system to notice parts who may want to lose weight.

What is your sense of how many of your parts would like to lose weight? Add these parts to your parts list.

_____

Check in with those parts and ask what they're hoping to achieve with weight loss. Describe their response.

_____

_____

_____

_____

_____

_____

What would your Self like to say to these parts?

_____

_____

_____

_____

_____

Some of their goals may be absolutely understandable. Life *is easier* in a smaller body for numerous reasons. But some of their goals may be fantasy. Many parts tend to believe that weight loss is *the* thing that fixes everything. Quite simply, it isn't. Spend time getting to know these parts and let them see that Self isn't concerned about size.

Let's Talk About Grief

One of the pieces of developing body respect that isn't often discussed is the experience of grief. Most likely, your parts have an image of what they want your body to look like. They may have had this image for years, even decades. You may have worked extremely hard to achieve this image, and you may have succeeded. But most likely, the body that your parts want you to be in isn't realistic. And it's *really difficult* to face and accept that. Our parts experience real grief when they realize that you are no longer working toward that image and that body won't be achieved. It's incredibly important to recognize, listen to, and validate that grief. This may be something to work through in therapy, if that's available to you.

Take a moment to check in with your system and notice any and all parts who are carrying grief about your body. Describe them here, and add them to your parts list.

_____

_____

_____

_____

_____

_____

_____

Additional Suggestions

Working toward body respect is often the most difficult piece of this work, but I wholeheartedly believe it can be done. Continue getting to know your parts and approaching them and your body with Self-energy. And here are a few additional suggestions:

- Monitor your social media.

- Do not follow anyone focusing on dieting, weight loss, or extreme exercise (the "no pain, no gain" gym bros).

- Do not follow anyone who posts before and after photos.

- Do follow people of all shapes, sizes, and colors—especially those who look like you!

- Do follow people who focus on Intuitive Eating, body neutrality, body acceptance, body liberation, and body positivity.

- Find others (either on social media or in real life) who are ditching diets and working toward body respect.

- Do not bond with others over dieting and body hatred—let them know this is a conversation you're no longer willing to have.

CHAPTER 9

Putting It All Together for Self-Led Eating

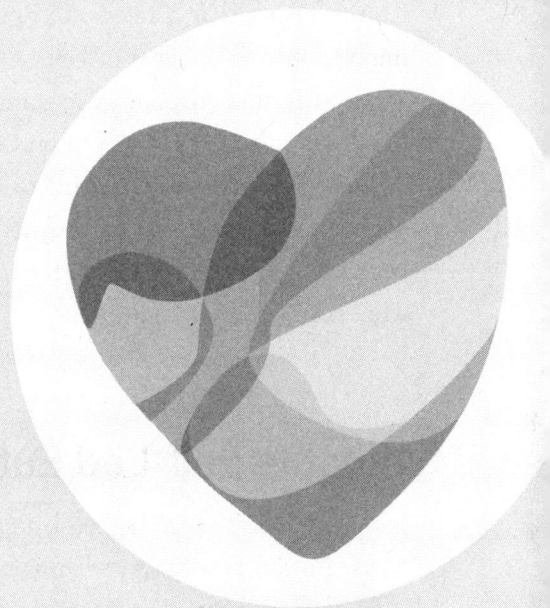

By this point, you've gotten to know your Self as well as many of your parts. You have a better understanding of your eating system, how it works, and why your parts use or restrict food the way they do. You're also beginning to develop respect for and connection to your body and are starting to nourish it in the ways that it needs. Congratulations—you've done a *lot* of work! And you've got the most important tools under your belt.

In this final chapter, we're going to dive into what Self-led eating looks like and how to get there. You'll also create a game plan on how to continue your progress, and we'll wrap up some loose ends. But most importantly, I'm going to give you a step-by-step process that guides you through what to do every time you turn to food. This will help you notice if you're heading to food out of hunger or because of a part; connect with parts when they're turning you to food in the moment; and discover what your body is hungry for.

What Is Self-Led Eating?

Just as the term suggests, Self-led eating refers to eating in a way that is guided by Self instead of by parts. As you now know, when your parts are running the show, they're using or restricting food in ways that are protective of themselves and other parts. Although this serves a purpose for them, it often leads to other difficulties and is not in the best interest of your body.

Conversely, Self approaches food with calmness and curiosity. Self has no agenda other than nourishing your body and also just enjoying a meal! Your core Self wants your parts—and your body—to be happy and healthy. It wants you to eat intuitively and also enjoyably. Self wants you to feel free and flexible with food and doesn't want to follow external food rules—because it doesn't need to.

All of that sounds great, doesn't it? Now that you have an idea of what Self-led eating looks like, it's time to talk about the actual eating process. When you notice wanting food, this obviously may be your body telling you it's hungry. However, as you very well know, eating often has nothing to do with hunger. Thanks to the work you've been doing in getting to know your parts, you now know more about why your parts turn you to food. Despite all this information, it still may be tough to know if you're truly hungry or if a part is leading you to food. And you may still have difficulty connecting with your eating parts in the moments when they're heading for the kitchen. That's completely understandable—this is often the hardest part of the work! And it's what we'll be talking about now.

What to Do When You're Heading for Food

This section walks you through checking in with your hunger cues, connecting with the part(s) that's leading you to food (if you're not actually hungry), and deciding what to eat. You'll notice that a large part of this process is what you already did in chapter 6 when you unblended from your firefighters. A condensed version of this eating guide is also available at http://www.newharbinger.com/57286—feel free to print it out and keep it nearby.

Step 1: Ask yourself, *Am I hungry?*

- With your Hunger Rating Scale nearby, check in with your body and notice your hunger level. (If you don't find the rating scale useful, that's fine—just do your best to tune into your body and recognize your hunger level. Or, if you're someone who tends to be aware of their hunger cues, just skip the rating scale.)

- If you're having difficulty noticing your hunger level, you may have a blocking part in the way. Walk away from the food and get curious about why you're having difficulty connecting to your body right now. Try to notice the part who's blocking your connection and get to know that part using the Getting to Know a Protector Part worksheet or meditation.

Step 2: If the answer is *Yes, I'm hungry enough to eat!*

- Tune into your body and consider what you're hungry for. What sounds good? Think about the taste, texture, and temperature of different foods, and do your best to find a food that sounds satisfying to your body.

- Tune into your parts and consider what they're hungry for as well. They get to eat what they enjoy too! However, sometimes our parts want food that our body doesn't want or that you know won't sit well with you. The part who wants this food is likely a part who is excited about food or maybe wants food as a reward. You have a few options here. Just be sure that you're approaching this part with a lot of Self-energy:

  - Get curious with this part and see if it's protecting another part. It may be trying to comfort or reward another part with food.

  - Let the part know that it can eat whatever it wants internally, meaning you won't actually eat, but it can imagine itself eating in its internal world.

· Remind the part that you're an adult now and you're trying to focus on what your body needs. Ask if it can give you the space to respect your body and eat what your body is asking for.

· Discuss a compromise with your part. Let it know that your Self wants it to be happy and that you're okay with eating what it wants, but let's eat it mindfully (see below).

Step 3: If the answer is *I'm not physically hungry—a part is definitely leading me to food.*

- Leave the room. It's much easier to connect to your parts when you aren't staring at their favorite food. Find somewhere quiet where you can check in with yourself.

- Ask the part to take a couple of steps back from you so that you can notice it and connect with it.

- Find your Self-energy. Let the part know that you're open and curious toward it, and that you'd love to offer your help. Unblend from any other parts who are present.

- Ask the part what's going on for it right now, and what led it to wanting food. Listen and validate the part.

- If you have time, get to know the part by using all of the steps from your Getting to Know a Protector Part worksheet or with the help of a meditation.

- Ask the part how you can be helpful to it. Ask what it would need to feel calmer. Do your best to give it what it needs.

- Thank the part for all it does for you.

- Make the commitment to check in with the part later in the day or the next day to see how it's doing.

Try this process a couple of times and reflect on it here.

What was it like to check in prior to eating?

_____

_____

_____

What did you notice about your body? Your parts?

_____

_____

_____

What was difficult about this process?

_____

_____

_____

What might be helpful for you to do the next time you try this?

_____

_____

_____

_____

_____

Eating Mindfully

Eating mindfully means really slowing down, using all your senses during the eating process, and checking in with your body while you're eating. To eat more mindfully, follow these steps:

- Before you begin eating, notice your hunger cues. (If you aren't hungry enough to eat, check in with whatever part is leading you to food.) Focus closely on the food on your plate, noticing its colors and aromas.

- While you're eating, be sure that you're chewing your food slowly and taking your time to eat. Continue to notice the colors and aromas of your food, and also notice the texture and the temperature. Try to find every ingredient that you know is in your food.

Continually check in with your satisfaction levels. How is your body responding to this food? How are your parts? Is it enjoyable and satisfying? If not, does it make sense to stop eating and find something else that sounds more appealing to your body and your parts? Check in with your fullness cues (using the Hunger Rating Scale) and try to stop eating at a 6. Notice any parts who may be trying to convince you to stop eating before this number or to continue eating past this number.

- After eating, notice how your body is feeling in response to this food. Did it sit well? Was it satisfying? Make a note of this information to help determine if you'd like to eat this food again. Check in with your parts and let them see how your body responded to this food.

Try this process a couple of times and reflect on it here.

What was is like to eat mindfully?

_____

_____

_____

What did you notice about the eating process?

_____

_____

_____

What was difficult about eating mindfully?

_____

_____

_____

What might be helpful for you to try the next time?

_____

_____

_____

_____

_____

_____

When Your Parts Won't Let You Check In

While reading this section, you may have many parts saying, "Yes! I'm going to do that whole check-in process every time I eat!" And lo and behold, a week goes by, and you haven't checked in once. You haven't even thought about it. That could be due to the fact that this is still a very new process for you, and it takes time to make it a habit. You can put a reminder on your phone or a Post-it on the fridge—anything to cue you to check in before eating.

Sometimes you may hear yourself say, _Eh—I'll do that whole check-in thing next time. I just really want to eat right now._ These are likely what I call "I don't care" parts speaking. They make you believe that you're not that invested in this process, that doing it isn't a big deal, or that it's just a waste of time. These are protective parts to get to know. In general, these are parts who are fearful of the check-in process and worry that they may do it wrong, that another part will take away the food they love, or that parts who feel shame about eating will come up. If you notice these parts, just add them to your parts list and get to know them like you would any other protector.

It's not easy to check in with yourself regularly when you're heading for food. If you haven't been checking in with yourself for years or even decades, you can't expect to do it perfectly right out of the gate. Do your best! At first, shoot for a reasonable goal—even once a week is a good starting point. Then once you've got that down, add another time. And another. And another.

Developing a Regular Parts Practice

In addition to checking in with your body and your parts prior to eating, it's *really* important to develop a practice of checking in with your parts as frequently as you're able. I'm guessing you've met quite a few parts by now, and your parts list is probably still quite long—try not to be overwhelmed! We all have dozens and dozens of parts, and it takes a lot of time to get to know them. Remember that you won't be getting to know all your parts. We have many parts in our system that are in the background just doing their thing and not causing any concerns. You likely won't meet these parts, and that's okay.

In this section, we're going to talk about how to create a regular parts practice and what to expect during that process. Let me say up front that you will *not* be checking in with every part you meet every day for the rest of your life. Please don't expect that of yourself. Generally speaking, the IFS community recommends that you check in with a part you've gotten to know every day for three weeks. This is especially important with exiles. You definitely want to make sure that your exiled parts know you're there to help them if they need you, and this consistent process helps build trust.

Creating Your Practice

As with many things, there is no right way to do this, and everyone does it differently. You may want to try a few different things and see what sticks. The most important thing is to create a practice that is realistic and sustainable for you. It's also vital to do this practice consistently, at least in the beginning. If you're checking in with your parts only once a month, they're not going to develop much trust in you. The more frequently you can do this, the better. Once more of your parts know you and see you being more present in your life, the less they'll need formal check-ins (except with your exiles—you always want to check in with them after you've met them).

For most people, choosing a time of day that lends itself to a check-in is a great way to start. Start by committing five or ten minutes to the process. It can also be helpful to pair the check-in process with another activity that lends itself to introspection, such as walking or meditating. It's also very helpful to have a journal handy to note who you've spoken to, where you noticed them, and if they'd like you to check in with them again.

Once you've determined a time and manner of check-in that works for you, here are some guidelines to follow:

- Take some deep breaths and turn your attention inward.

- Notice how open your heart feels. Invite in your calm, compassionate Self-energy, and ask parts to settle back and notice you.

- Begin to notice your parts. You can do this by asking who's there and waiting for an answer, or noticing sensations in your body. Invite these parts to tell you anything they would like you to know. If you're limited on time, let them know that you don't have as much time as you usually do, and that you'll make a note of getting back to them later if they need you to.

- If there's a particular part you'd like to check in with, ask if that part is here with you now. If you have difficulty accessing it, think about where the part was when you connected with it last; for example, was it hanging out at the beach? Or try to recall how it showed up for you physically when you connected with it.

- Once you've found the part, ask how it's doing and if there's anything it would like you to know. Remind it that you are a resource for it and that you'll be checking in with it again.

- If you've been checking in with this part consistently for a while now, ask if it still needs these check-ins. It likely won't. Just let it know that it can always get your attention if it needs you in the future.

- Use a journal to jot down which part you spoke with, where it showed up for you, and if it would like to speak with you again. These can be detailed notes of your conversation or just quick notes to jog your memory. There are also books and journals you can purchase to help with this process. Those resources are listed in the back of this book.

What to Expect from This Practice

Checking in doesn't always go smoothly, at least initially. You may encounter some of these common difficulties:

- Sometimes you can't find a particular part you've gotten to know in order to check in with it. It may just be off doing its thing—that's fine. Sometimes, though, a part is blocking your access to another part out of concern. Gently check to see if this is happening. And sometimes, there are just too many other parts who need your attention.

- When you unburden parts, you may never see them again even if you try to connect with them. Sometimes our parts are so relieved by dropping their burdens that they run off into the sunset, never to be seen again. They're now an integrated part of your system, and they're doing fine.

- You'll likely have parts who are such an important part of your system that you're in contact with them a lot. Some people have CEOs who play a big role in their system, and your Self and this part can work together as a team.

Your Game Plan

At this point, you have every tool in your toolbox. Congratulations! You may be wondering where to go from here. Keep in mind that there is no right way to continue with your progress. Everyone's path is different, as are everyone's needs.

There are many activities you can engage in to help you continue this work, and I've listed my recommendations below. This list is in no particular order (although the first recommendation is the most important one!), and some of these activities will be more necessary for you than others.

Continue getting to know your parts. *This is the most important piece.* By now, you have a good idea of the parts who run your eating system and why. Continue using your worksheets and the prerecorded meditations to get to know these parts more fully.

Build trust between your Self and your parts by maintaining a regular check-in practice and by returning to parts who you've met (especially exiles) for at least three weeks after meeting them.

Continue to meet your exiles. Remember that these are the parts your eating-restricting parts are protecting, and once they feel witnessed and validated, protectors can begin to soften. If at all possible, please work with an IFS therapist or practitioner who can help you to unburden your exiles. See the list of resources at the back of the book to help you find one.

Work toward body respect by getting to know the parts of you who carry negative thoughts and beliefs about your body. Remind yourself that Self does not believe there is anything wrong with your body and Self is not trying to fix or change it.

Continue to educate yourself on diet culture, noticing the messages that your parts learned and still carry about bodies, beauty, and thinness. Check out the resource list at the back of the book for information on books, podcasts, and websites that will be helpful in this process.

Develop a stronger connection to your body by getting to know the parts of you who may be blocking it. Use your IFS skills to get curious about these parts and your IE skills to notice and understand more about what your body is telling you.

Take a moment to reflect on these recommendations before creating your own game plan. Your plan will change as your work progresses, so consider it a living document. It may be helpful to choose one or two activities to focus on at a time. Once you feel as though you've made sufficient progress, choose another one or two. For example, the information on diet culture may be brand-new to you. It might be helpful to work on learning more about its impact and get to know the parts of you who continue to carry its messaging. Once you feel as though enough of your parts have absorbed this information, move on to another activity, such as working toward body respect.

The worksheet that follows is also available at http://www.newharbinger.com/57286 for you to print out when you need to update your plan.

My Game Plan

Which activities feel the most important to me at this time?

- ☐ Getting to know my parts (this one should always be on the list!)

- ☐ Building trust between my Self and my parts

- ☐ Meeting my exiles

- ☐ Working toward body respect

- ☐ Educating myself on diet culture

- ☐ Developing a stronger connection to my body

What are the common themes I've noticed with my parts?

_____

_____

_____

_____

What parts would I like to explore at this point?

_____

_____

_____

How am I feeling toward food? How (if at all) would I like that to change?

_____

_____

_____

_____

How am I feeling toward my body? How (if at all) would I like that to change?

_____

_____

_____

_____

What do I notice about my progress so far?

_____

_____

_____

_____

_____

_____

Here's at least one thing that I feel good about: (Feel free to list more than one!)

_____

_____

_____

_____

_____

_____

_____

Concluding Thoughts

You have no doubt done significant work on your system thus far, and I'm confident that you've noticed at least a small shift in your relationship toward food and your body. I find that for most people, change is subtle—until it's not. Since you aren't working on behavior change, you may not see progress initially. But then one day, you'll just notice a shift. Things feel a little easier with food. A behavior you've tried so hard to change in the past seems to happen without your even trying. This is the way it tends to happen.

A few concluding thoughts:

- Remember, this is a marathon, not a sprint. You'll be in contact with your parts for the rest of your life—you don't need to get to know all of them right now. Encourage your parts to be patient.

- We're constantly swimming in messages about bodies, weight, and food that likely impact our parts. You will probably always have parts who think about weight loss, want to diet, or restrict your food to some degree. But you now have the ability to notice and unblend from them so that they don't take over. You can also remind these parts that your Self knows you and your body are valuable just the way you are.

- Remember that it's okay for food to still be comforting. As you read in chapter 1, food *is* nurturing and enjoyable, and you don't need to give it up completely. But, if you continue to work with your emotional eating parts, you will continue to notice a lessening of that drive. And you, again, will have the ability to notice and unblend from them. If they still really want the food, that's okay! Eat it with them mindfully, enjoy it, and move on. Sometimes food *is* still the thing that works.

- The goal isn't to be Self-led all the time. That's impossible. Don't expect yourself to check in every single time you eat—that takes more time and attention than most of us have. That's okay! The goal is to have more of your Self present and have space from your parts so that you're better able to notice and unblend from them when they arise.

- Try to find support. If it feels safe to you, talk to people around you about what you're working toward and why. Ask for what you need from them. This might be asking them to limit their discussions of dieting, not commenting on their or others' bodies, or even keeping certain foods away from you until you feel ready to face them. Sometimes, the entire topic of food and bodies needs to be off-limits. You have the right to ask for this.

I hope that your parts are feeling very proud of what you've accomplished thus far. *This is really difficult work,* and I'm so very happy that you've taken the time to do it. You deserve it! And you deserve peace and freedom with food and your body. I'm honored to have walked this road with you.

Acknowledgments

I've wanted to write a book for years, and I'm so incredibly thankful that I waited this long. A book I would've written ten years ago would *not* be the book you're reading now. And it honestly wouldn't have been helpful. To get to the point of writing *this* book, I had to meet many people along the way. And those are the people I would like to thank now.

I need to start with Sue, my friend and colleague, who became my coworker in the 2010s and spoke in this strange language of parts. Sue, had you not offered to give me a free IFS session, I have no idea if I would've found my way to this world. I'm so grateful to you for that.

Next up were my IFS Level 1 trainers, Ralph and Ann, who created a warm, informative space to learn a model that was intimidating to my system and yet resonated so deeply. I've had numerous trainers since that Level 1, but on the days that I believe I'm being a really good therapist, I know I'm channeling one of you.

I next need to thank Tammy Sollenberger, who graciously allowed me to be on her well-known podcast, *The One Inside*, and introduced me to her book "people." This led me to the amazing Jane Gerhard, my first editor and guide, who made me start to think I actually had something to say. Thanks so much, Jane, for your insight, your support, and your ability to ask questions that made me dig a little deeper.

A huge thanks to Jed Bickman, of New Harbinger, who thought this book was a good idea and moved it along faster than I anticipated. And to my editor Madison Davis, who offered great advice in a supportive, positive way.

To my friends and family who continually asked how this project was going, knowing that I don't tend to offer information on such things but of course would love to share about it.

And finally, my deepest gratitude to all the clients I've had the honor of working with. You've been a constant inspiration, and you've taught me far more than I've ever taught you.

Glossary of IFS Terms

You can refer back to this glossary while reading the book, until these terms become second nature.

Blended: When a part has merged with you and taken control of the wheel.

Burdens: The extreme thoughts and beliefs that your parts carry. These have generally resulted from your experiences of trauma and other emotional injuries.

Exiles: The parts of you who are carrying burdens. They tend to be young parts and may be stuck in the past.

Firefighters: Protective parts who are impulsive and reactive. Their goal is generally to completely numb your system.

Managers: Protective parts who are proactive and work to keep your life running.

Parts: The subpersonalities who make up your system and run the show at different times. There are no bad parts. All of your parts are doing their best to protect you.

Polarizations: When parts want opposite things, such as a binge eating part and a restrictive part.

Unblending: The process of separating from your parts so that you can offer them Self-energy.

Unburdening: The process by which we help our parts let go of the burdens they carry, which allows them to return to their original intentions.

Updating: The process by which we tell our parts our present age and show them our current lives.

Resource List

Books

Catanzaro, J. 2024. *Unburdened Eating: Healing Your Relationships with Food and Your Body Using an Internal Family Systems (IFS) Approach.* Eau Claire, WI: Bridge City Books.

Engeln, R. 2018. *Beauty Sick: How the Cultural Obsession with Appearance Hurts Girls and Women.* New York: Harper Paperbacks.

Gay, R. 2018. *Hunger: A Memoir of (My) Body.* New York: Harper Perennial.

Gordon, A. 2021. *What We Don't Talk About When We Talk About Fat.* Boston: Beacon Press.

Gordon, A. 2023. *"You Need to Lose Weight" and 19 Other Myths About Fat People.* Boston: Beacon Press.

Kinavey, H., and D. Sturtevant. 2022. *Reclaiming Body Trust: A Path to Healing and Liberation.* New York: TarcherPerigee.

Kopald, S. 2023. *Self-Led: Living a Connected Life with Yourself and with Others.* Exploration Services, LLC.

Matz, J., A. Pershing, and C. Harrison. 2024. *The Emotional Eating, Chronic Dieting, Binge Eating, and Body Image Workbook: A Trauma-Informed, Weight-Inclusive Approach to Make Peace with Food and Reduce Body Shame.* Eau Claire, WI: PESI Publishing.

Pershing, A., and C. Turner. 2018. *Binge Eating Disorder: The Journey to Recovery and Beyond.* New York: Routledge.

Schwartz, R. 2021. *No Bad Parts: Healing Trauma and Restoring Wholeness with the Internal Family Systems Model.* Boulder, CO: Sounds True.

Schwartz, R. 2023. *Introduction to Internal Family Systems.* Boulder, CO: Sounds True.

Schwartz, R. 2024. *The Internal Family Systems Workbook: A Guide to Discover Your Self and Heal Your Parts.* Boulder, CO: Sounds True.

Sollenberger, T. 2022. *The One Inside: Thirty Days to Your Authentic Self*. Phoenix: Pure Carbon Publishing.

Strings, S. 2019. *Fearing the Black Body*. New York: University Press.

Taylor, S. R. 2021. *The Body Is Not an Apology: The Power of Radical Self-Love*. 2nd ed. Oakland, CA: Berrett-Koehler Publishers.

Taylor, S. R. 2021. *Your Body Is Not an Apology Workbook: Tools for Living Radical Self-Love*. Oakland, CA: Berrett-Koehler Publishers.

Tribole, E., and E. Resch. 2020. *Intuitive Eating: A Revolutionary Anti-Diet Approach*. 4th ed. New York: St. Martin's Essentials.

Tribole, E., and E. Resch. 2025. *The Intuitive Eating Workbook: Ten Principles for Nourishing a Healthy Relationship with Food*. 2nd ed. Oakland, CA: New Harbinger Publications.

West, C. 2021. *We All Have Parts: An Illustrated Guide to Healing Trauma with Internal Family Systems*. Eau Claire, WI: PESI Publishing.

Journaling Workbooks

Glass, M. 2016. *Daily Parts Meditation Practice: A Journey of Embodied Integration for Clients and Therapists*. The Listen3r.

Hedman, T. 2023. *Journal Back to Self: A 13-Week Internal Family Systems Guided Exploration*. Hedman Wellness Services.

Podcasts

Atwood, A. *The Full Plate Podcast*.

Daniels, K. *The Emotional Eating (and Everything Else) Podcast*.

Dillon, J. D. *Find Your Food Voice*.

Gordon, A., and M. Hobbes. *Maintenance Phase*.

Harrison, C. *Food Psych Podcast*.

Previte, S., and J. Werner *What the Actual Fork*.

Scritchfield, R. *Body Kindness.*

Sole-Smith, V. *Burnt Toast*

Sollenberger, T. *The One Inside: An Internal Family Systems (IFS) Podcast.*

Websites

Association for Size Diversity and Health: https://asdah.org/

The IFS Institute: https://ifs-institute.com/

Intuitive Eating: https://www.intuitiveeating.org/

National Eating Disorder Association: https://www.nationaleatingdisorders.org/

Websites to Help You Find a Therapist

The IFS Institute lists therapists who have completed official Level 1 IFS trainings. Definitely start there! If you're unable to find someone, try the other options listed and also search for IFS or IFS-informed therapists who specialize in eating disorders or disordered eating.

The IFS Institute: https://ifs-institute.com/practitioners
   (For practitioners in Canada, visit IFSCA: https://ifsca.ca/ifs-directory/)

American Association for Marriage and Family Therapy: https://www.aamft.org/Directories/Find_a_Therapist.aspx

American Psychological Association: https://locator.apa.org/

Good Therapy: https://www.goodtherapy.org/

Psychology Today: https://www.psychologytoday.com/us

Therapist.com: https://therapist.com/

Therapy Den: https://www.therapyden.com/

ZenCare: https://zencare.co/

References

Businesswire. 2023. "United States Weight Loss & Diet Control Market Report 2023."
https://www.businesswire.com/news/home/.

Harrison, C. 2021. *Anti-Diet: Reclaim Your Time, Money, Well-Being, and Happiness Through Intuitive Eating.* New York: Little, Brown Spark.

Patton, G. C., R. Selzer, C. Coffey, J. B. Carlin, and R. Wolfe. 1999. "Onset of Adolescent Eating Disorders: Population Based Cohort Study Over 3 Years." *British Medical Journal* 318 (7186): 765–768.

Schwartz, R. 1995. *Internal Family Systems.* New York: Guilford Press.

Tribole, E. and E. Resch. 2020. *Intuitive Eating: A Revolutionary Anti-Diet Approach.* 4th ed. New York: St. Martin's Essentials.

Tribole, E. and E. Resch. 2025. *The Intuitive Eating Workbook: Ten Principles for Nourishing a Healthy Relationship with Food.* 2nd ed. Oakland, CA: New Harbinger Publications.

Kimberly M. Daniels, PsyD, is a clinical psychologist who has specialized in treating disordered eating for more than twenty years. She is a certified level 2 trained Internal Family Systems (IFS) therapist, an approved IFS consultant, and a certified Intuitive Eating counselor. She is passionate about empowering women, and helping them to heal their relationship with food and their bodies once and for all. She lives near Hartford, CT.

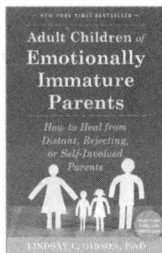

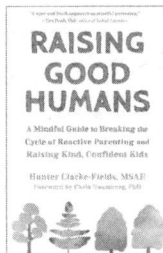

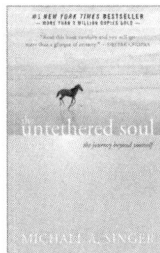

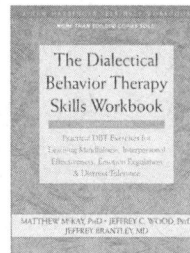

Did you know there are **free tools** you can download for this book?

Free tools are things like **worksheets**, **guided meditation exercises**, and **more** that will help you get the most out of your book.

You can download free tools for this book— whether you bought or borrowed it, in any format, from any source—from the New Harbinger website. All you need is a NewHarbinger.com account. Just use the URL provided in this book to view the free tools that are available for it. Then, click on the "download" button for the free tool you want, and follow the prompts that appear to log in to your NewHarbinger.com account and download the material.

You can also save the free tools for this book to your **Free Tools Library** so you can access them again anytime, just by logging in to your account! Just look for this button on the book's free tools page.

+ Save this to my free tools library

If you need help accessing or downloading free tools, visit **newharbinger.com/faq** or contact us at **customerservice@newharbinger.com**.